CLEAN LIVING

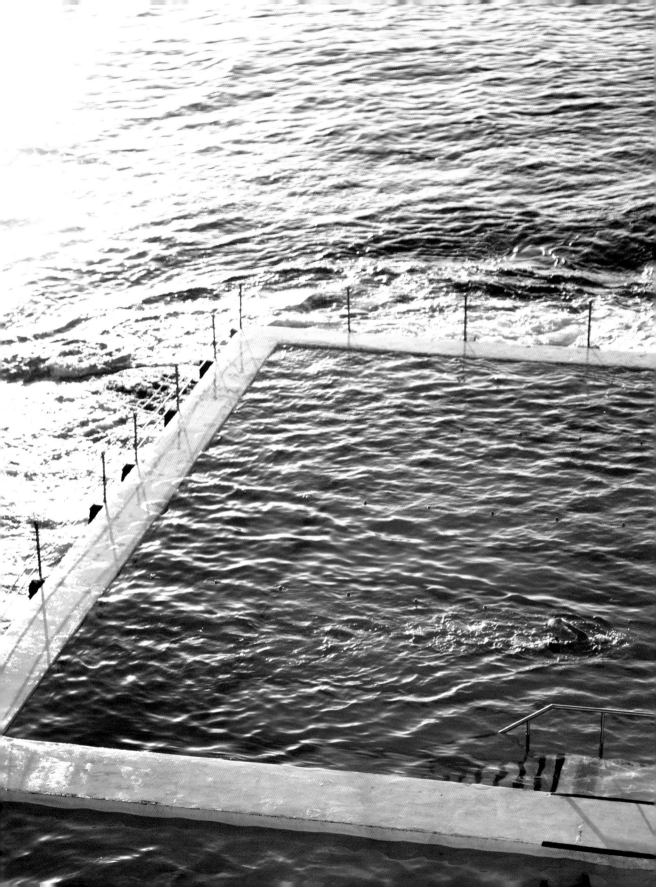

To Manny
MARVEY *on your birthday*

LUKE HINES AND SCOTT GOODING

CLEAN LIVING

A 3-WEEK HEALTHY LIFESTYLE PLAN TO HELP YOU CHANGE YOUR LIFE

love Granny
X

hachette
AUSTRALIA

IMPORTANT NOTE TO READERS: Although every effort has been made to ensure that the contents of this book are accurate, it must not be treated as a substitute for qualified medical advice. Always consult a qualified medical practitioner. Neither the authors nor the publisher can be held responsible for any loss or claim arising out of the use, or misuse, of the suggestions made or the failure to take professional medical advice.

hachette
AUSTRALIA

Published in Australia and New Zealand in 2013
by Hachette Australia
(an imprint of Hachette Australia Pty Limited)
Level 17, 207 Kent Street, Sydney NSW 2000
www.hachette.com.au

10 9 8 7 6 5 4 3

National Library of Australia
Cataloguing-in-Publication data

Hines, Luke, author.
Clean living / Luke Hines and Scott Gooding.

ISBN 978 0 7336 3169 6 (paperback)

Health.
Physical fitness.
Nutrition.

Other authors: Gooding, Scott, author.

613

Cover design and text design by Liz Seymour
Typeset in PMN Caecillia by Agave Creative
Photography by Steve Brown
Food preparation by Tracey Meharg
Styling by Trish Heagerty
Photography with permission of Waverley Council
Printed in China by Toppan Leefung Printing Limited

CONTENTS

Foreword

One of the best feelings in life is that one you get when you connect with like-minded people – knowledge-seeking, enthusiastic, practical people who understand the uncomplicated keys to an extraordinary life, and are happy to share them. Reading this book reminded me exactly of how I felt when I first met Luke and Scott. *Clean Living* reflects the refreshing and unique energy that the boys exude day in and day out. Luke and Scott will be the first ones to tell you that it isn't difficult to look and feel your best, you just need to follow some pretty basic guidelines. In this book they show us what to eat – or, more importantly in this day and age, what not to eat – and introduce us to a variety of exercises that remind us how fun and spontaneous a healthy lifestyle can be.

Now, it's no secret that I'm into everything related to health and wellness, so I'm honoured to be able to share a few words about my personal connection to the boys. It all began on a little cooking show in which Luke and Scott were in the hot seat under all the pressure, and I was pretty much kicking back sharing a few tips here and a few tips there, and enjoying their creations in the kitchen. However, the tables have since turned and now I'm the one under the pump – training like a man on a mission with the boys' encouraging guidance. My family and I have developed a friendship with Luke and Scott, and they have indeed helped me with my training by introducing me to a whole new world of engaging exercise. They both walk the walk and talk the talk of optimum health, and I firmly believe that it's wise to take advice and learn from people who are living proof of what they advocate. I often ask people: 'How healthy is your health adviser? Would you rather take advice from someone with a degree, who is overweight and has health problems, or do you look for direction from people who radiate energy and embody vigour?' I know my choice is the latter.

As personal trainers the fellas have probably heard all the excuses in the world as to why people haven't got time for their health, but I believe that time is all we *do* have and I'm sure most of us desire more quality time on this planet rather than less. So, summon your courage and let your excuses go, tell all your friends and family that you're going to make a commitment to being the best you can be and ask them for their support. Who knows, your choice to improve your lifestyle may well be the catalyst that motivates someone else to leap onto a similar path towards health and vitality. My favourite saying is, 'YOU have to be the change!'.

Clean Living contains crucial knowledge that's vital for the survival of our species and our planet. That may sound over-the-top, but in all seriousness it couldn't be closer to the truth. With obesity, diabetes, cardiovascular disease, cancer and countless other illnesses all on the rise, it most certainly is the time to begin taking the all-important steps towards a mindful lifestyle, and nutrition and exercise are an integral part of that journey. By following the boys' straightforward guidelines – fun exercise and some simple yet delicious recipes – you'll be well on your way!

My family and I have been following a paleolithic lifestyle for the last couple of years and our health has never been better, so I'm particularly proud of the boys' first offering in this space. I'm sure it won't be the last because, let's face it, healthy food is yummy food!

Keep cooking with love and laughter.

Pete Evans

Cookbook author, television presenter and award-winning chef

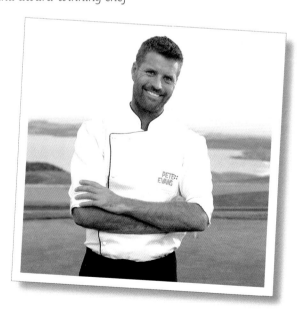

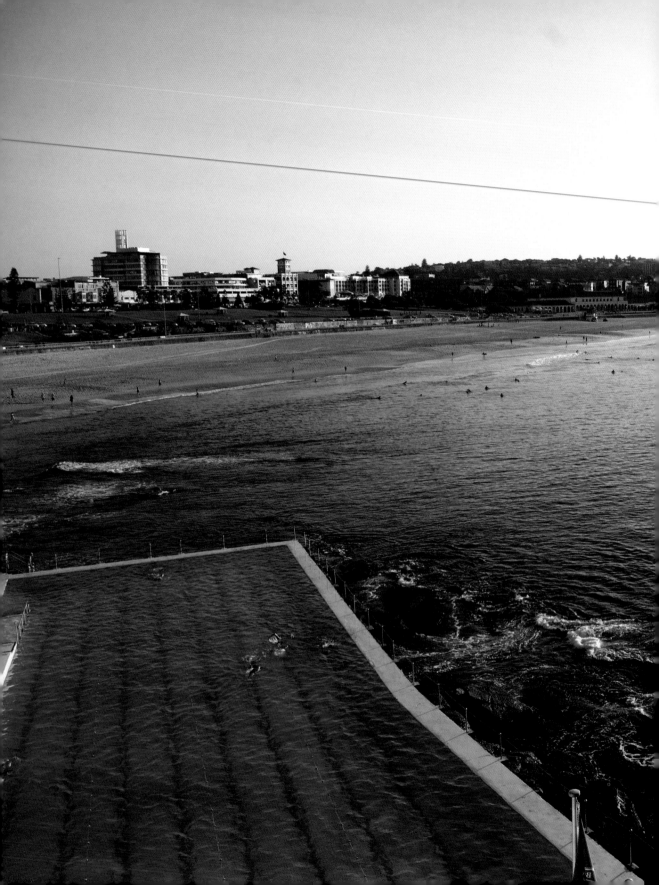

Let us introduce ourselves . . . .

We are two Bondi boys who believe strongly in a few simple things in life. These aren't things we can hold in our hands. They don't have a price tag or a use-by date. They're not expensive, or fancy. They are simple things within everyone's reach – things you can start working towards today and enjoy for the rest of your life. Wanna know what these things are? That's easy. They are a healthy body and a healthy mind. Pretty simple, huh? These two things are the basis of our way of life, a way of life we are lucky enough to be able to share with you.

This book, *Clean Living*, was born from our once-in-a-lifetime experience cooking healthy food on the hit series *My Kitchen Rules*. We were given a phenomenal opportunity to share our message of health and wellness with people all around the country. Having generated such interest in our way of life, we felt it was important to use our public profile to educate and inspire Australians to make positive life choices. So, we want to share with you a lifestyle program that is easy to follow, enjoyable each day, and sustainable long-term – one you will be able to stick with for the rest of your life.

We are passionate about living well because we have seen the results first hand, not only in ourselves but in our clients, through our personal training businesses. Simple adjustments to the way we move our bodies and the way we eat can translate into dramatic results both inside and out. When you start the *Clean Living* lifestyle program, you will see and feel a difference in just a short time.

We subscribe to the principles of the 'paleolithic lifestyle', believing that we should eat as close as we can to the way our hunter-gatherer ancestors did. That means a diet rich in a variety of sources of animal protein, good fats, nuts, seeds and fresh fruit and vegetables, with no grains and no processed sugar. Food is fuel – the wood we need to keep the fire burning – so it should be real, whole and natural. It should nourish us, but it should also be delicious. We want to smash the myth that to eat clean you have to sacrifice flavour, and in this book we prove that healthy food can also be *tasty* food.

It is vital that we understand what goes into our bodies – so we'll give you lots of high-quality nutritional information, explained in a way that is easy to understand.

We'll also suggest meal plans, give you tips to help you make smart choices when you're shopping, cooking and eating, and share fantastic recipes to make your kitchen rule! You'll be whipping up our healthy meals sooner than you can give yourself a perfect score for healthy living. And what's even better is that it's easier than you think. We bring cooking back to basics, so everyone can achieve a healthy lifestyle – there are no excuses not to enjoy fresh and healthy meals at home.

Our paleo philosophy is also reflected in our beliefs about movement. Humans used to hunt and gather, but today many of us lead sedentary lives. We believe that we should move our bodies like our ancestors did millions of years ago – pulling, pushing, lifting, dragging, twisting, running and jumping. These are primal movements, functional and effective, and they form the basis of our work-out program. We want to free you from the constraints of traditional methods of exercise and help you to move the way you were designed to move. Following our program will transform your body into a well-oiled, high-performance machine. You'll be fit and strong and feel amazing – and the results will be long-lasting.

It's widely accepted that it takes us around twenty-one days to change a habit, so we've designed our meal and exercise plans to be the perfect three-week overhaul – exactly what you need to kickstart you into a new way of life. We hope the new habits you form will last well past this twenty-one-day period and become an everyday part of your life.

We don't offer gimmicks, cheats or expensive quick fixes – just science-based training that gets results, combined with nutritionally sound eating advice. Our program caters for everyone – from beginners all the way to advanced – because we want to prove that everyone can look and feel great, no matter what their fitness level or experience.

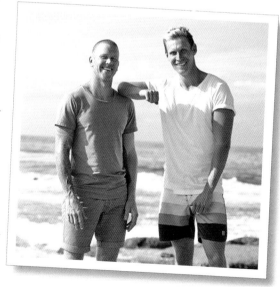

Life is all about choices. We all have the choice to be as fit and well as we can be. Living clean every day is easy, efficient, economical and sustainable – and all you need to do is follow the few easy principles we outline in this book. If we move our bodies and eat amazingly well, we feel fantastic – making us the best version of ourselves we can possibly be.

Luke & Scott x

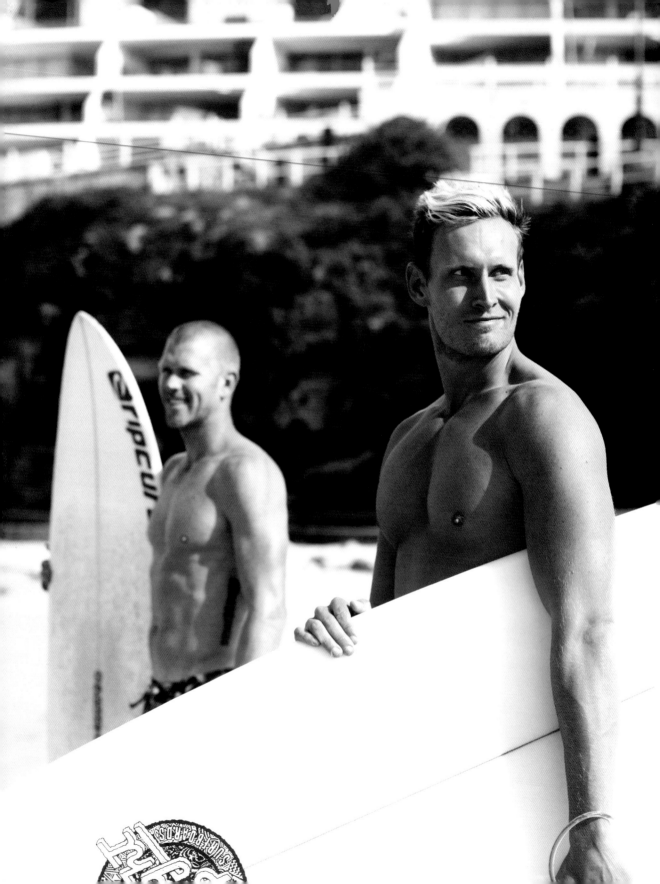

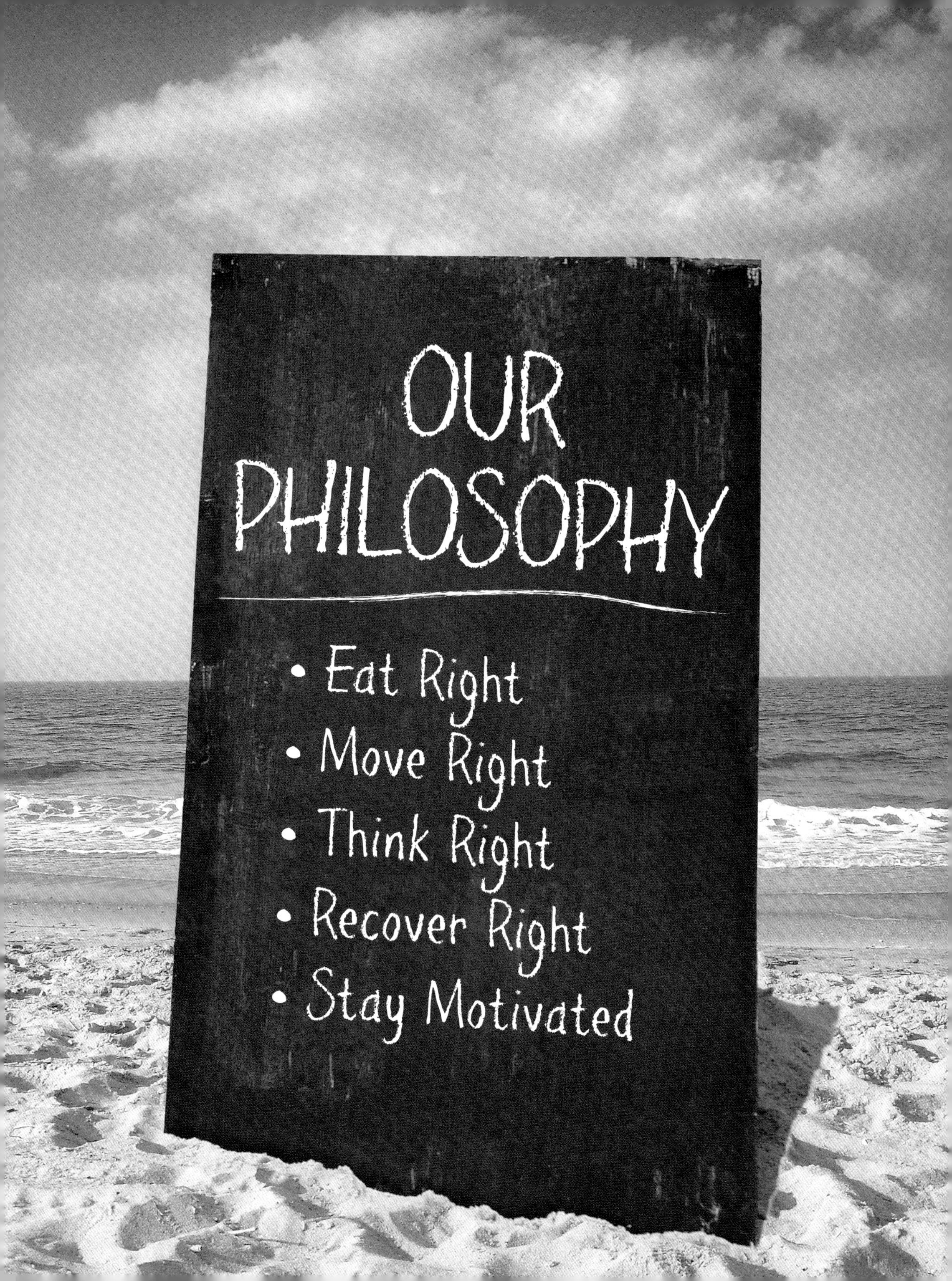
OUR
PHILOSOPHY
• Eat Right
• Move Right
• Think Right
• Recover Right
• Stay Motivated

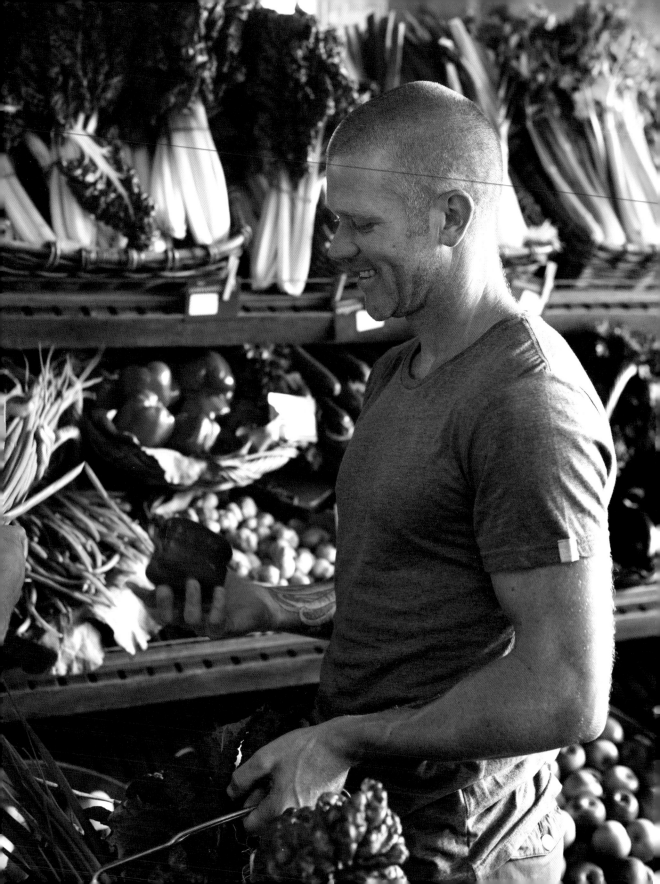

Eat Right

What we put into our bodies determines how we feel and how we perform. When you recognise the direct impact food has on your wellbeing, you will make smarter choices about what you eat. Imagine you bought a brand-new, top-of-its-class vehicle. You wouldn't fill it with crappy, low-quality petrol, would you? No, you would take great care of it and spend that little bit of extra time, care, attention and money on it, making sure you could enjoy it for a lifetime. Well, your body should be no different.

Our clients often tell us that their past experiences with healthy eating have been repetitive, boring and, even worse, bland. Clean eating doesn't have to be any of these things – and we can prove it! In fact, clean food is some of the most versatile, vibrant and delicious food you can enjoy. Our recipes offer an array of wonderful tastes – but they also provide you with all the nutrients you need to perform at your best.

If we understand what the various components of food do to our bodies, we can make conscious choices about what to eat, knowing how it will affect us. We recommend that you eat foods high in protein and good fats, choose your carbohydrates wisely, and avoid processed or refined sugars. Simple, easy and effective. We could write chapters and chapters on our beliefs about food, but we feel these four main components – protein, fats, carbohydrates and sugar – are really worth understanding. Let's look at them more closely.

Protein

Protein is vital for human survival – it forms the building blocks of our whole strength and recovery system. Put simply, protein is a combination of amino acids that help our body to repair muscle tissue, protect our skin, fight disease, give us energy and promote the correct hormone balance. There are two major types of amino acids: non-essential amino acids, manufactured by our bodies, and essential amino acids, found in our food. Not all forms of protein are created equal – some contain all the essential amino acids, and are therefore known as 'complete' proteins. Complete proteins include all animal sources of protein, as well as quinoa, which is a seed. Vegetable sources of protein contain only a few of the essential amino acids, and should be combined with other proteins. We recommend an eating plan high in protein. Our recipes use a variety of meats, including chicken and fish, as well as quinoa and other vegetable sources of protein.

Fats

Let's clear this up first off: there are good fats and there are bad fats. Every day we learn more and more about the role fats play in our diet – what fats we should be consuming, and why they are good for us – forcing us to rethink what we have been told for years.

These are the fats we recommend as part of our clean eating program:

Coconut fat

Coconuts are a true superfood. The whole coconut can be used, making it a great environmentally sustainable food crop. The flesh can be used for cooking, baking and smoothies, while the oil can be used for frying. We recommend coconut oil for frying, because its chemical structure remains consistent even when heated to high temperatures. It's also a wonderful source of energy.

Avocado fat

Avocados are packed full of mono-unsaturated fats, which are easily used by our bodies for energy. We all love avocado sliced over our breakfast on a Sunday morning, of course, and they're a fantastic fruit to add to salads, meat dishes and smoothies – but what most people don't know is that you can actually use avocado oil in your cooking. Found in all good supermarkets, it's a great alternative to the many different oils on the market and is awesome drizzled over a salad.

Animal fats

There's a lot we could learn from our prehistoric ancestors about how to eat meat. They used to eat almost every part of an animal, wasting nothing. Forget about trimming the fat off, or choosing skinless or fat-free cuts of meat – just eat the animal as it should be consumed, naturally. Animal fats are actually amazing sources of energy, and our bodies understand how to convert this fat into fuel.

Nut fats

Nuts are an excellent source of good fats. Packed full of vital omega-3 fatty acids, they give us long-term energy, aid weight loss, and are packed full of protein. Not only are they the quintessential food sourced from the land, they come in a range of flavours, colours and textures, which is great from a cook's perspective. Our recipes often include nuts, and we recommend you add them to your eating plan regularly.

Carbohydrates

Carbohydrates are a crucial part of the human diet – you can't live without them. They are an important source of energy and, in conjunction with protein, help us repair and grow. We do not recommend low-carb or no-carb diets. You can eat carbohydrates and stay lean, fit and healthy – you just need to consume them wisely. Carbohydrates can have a direct effect on your waistline, mood and energy levels, so you need to eat the right types in the right quantities. We don't prescribe a diet heavy in grains, rather one that is high in sweet potato, quinoa, buckwheat, amaranth, fresh fruit and seasonal vegetables – all of which are fantastic sources of carbohydrates. We look forward to exploring these ingredients with you in more detail in our recipes section.

Sugar

Low-sugar and no-sugar diets are popular at the moment, and for good reason. Studies have shown that fructose (an elemental sugar found in carbohydrates such as fruit) is harmful to our systems and causes many health problems, such as obesity and diabetes. Fructose inhibits the trigger that tells us we are 'full' and so it's not hard to see the causal link between a high fructose diet and weight gain. It is therefore necessary to be mindful of the amount of fructose in our diets. We are not advocating avoiding fruit, but we do suggest eating whole fruit rather than fruit juice, and avoiding copious amounts of fruit with high fructose levels, such as pears or grapes. Processed forms of sugar such as those found in cereals, breads, lollies, sweets, cakes and milk chocolate are definitely out – they offer no nutritional benefit, affect our energy levels dramatically, and can lead to unwanted weight gain and mood swings. Refined sugars are loaded with fructose and should be avoided. We sweeten our recipes with rice malt syrup rather than sugar. We also recommend that you avoid lactose, otherwise known as milk sugar. Cut out all the junk and see how good you look and feel.

Move Right

What does exercise mean to you? If we were to ask a roomful of people that question, we're confident we'd get a roomful of different answers – but they'd all involve movement of some description. Different forms of movement suit different people. Some people love running, for example, but it's definitely not for everyone. The key is to find the style of movement that works for you and makes you feel happy – only then will you be able to stick to your training program.

One thing we all have in common is that we don't move enough. Just cast your mind back to our ancestors, who roamed the earth for over 2 million years. They had to move to survive, had to forage, run, hunt, climb, build, swim, drag, push and pull, and periodically trek to more favourable regions. It's not a coincidence that we thrived and multiplied – it's because humans evolved to cope with these challenges. Our anatomy and physiology are proof of this. We have two different kinds of muscle fibre to help us respond appropriately to our environment – fast twitch fibres for when we need speed and power, and slow twitch fibres for steady movement requiring stamina and endurance. We have also developed an endocrine system that prepares us for fight or flight and regulates our energy consumption. There is no denying we are built to move – but our life today is sedentary.

Technology can improve our lives, but it also has a downside. Cars, trains, buses and planes allow us to travel long distances without effort. There's no need to hunt for foods – we can pick them up at the supermarket or even order them online. And whether we're working or relaxing, many of us spend huge parts of every day sitting in front of a screen. We are denying our primal nature, and it has serious consequences for our health. We've given up the habits formed over millions of years, and we've done it so quickly our bodies haven't had a chance to catch up. To restore the right balance, we need to get in touch with our primal side.

So what is primal training?

Primal training is functional training. It mimics everyday functions – the movements you make in daily life. The growth and popularity of intense cross-training programs is no accident. When you dissect these programs, you can see that they are made up of primal movements. As humans, we naturally gravitate to this approach – it makes the most of our bodies' innate skills and abilities, and we all like to do what we're good at. You don't necessarily need to sign up to your nearest gym, though – you can do a primal work-out in your lounge room, or at the park or the beach. In this book we've included our own three-week training program, which you can follow on your own or with a trainer (see page 136).

Our program is varied and challenging. It will help you to build every facet of fitness – strength, power, speed and endurance. This is very important, as building just one facet – strength alone, for example – can lead to overuse injuries, and you're also likely to grow bored with the narrow focus of your routine and give it up. The exercises we recommend use every part of the body, mimicking the movements our ancestors used every day, but adapting them to suit our modern way of life.

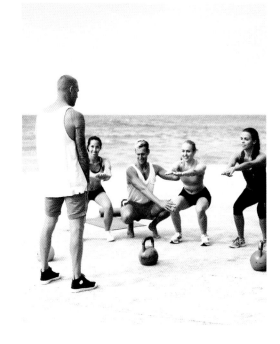

The exercises are based mainly on 'large compound movements' – movements involving more than one joint. (The squat is a good example of a compound movement, as it uses the hip, knee and ankle joints.) Exercises that require the use of multiple joints are preferable to isolated movements (such as a dumbbell bicep curl), because of the number of muscles that have to work in synergy. Remember: the more joints involved, the more muscles are activated. This also stresses and conditions your nervous system. We advocate compound, functional movements, as these will deliver a more complete fitness and get results more quickly.

These are great benefits, of course, but functional training has another important advantage. Compound movements may have their roots in strength training, but if you perform enough reps at the right tempo they become a form of aerobic training, too – killing two fitness birds with one stone. This means you can train for short periods of time but still reap the benefits of a good work-out. Short,

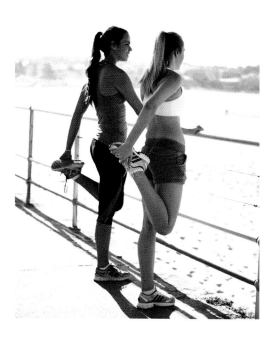

intense work-outs deliver more results than longer, less intense work-outs. This is the perfect scenario for us time-poor folk. Intense work-outs also promote the release of feel-good hormones. You'll know when they kick in. Test it for yourself: compare how you feel after a half-hour walk versus working out as hard as you can for ten minutes.

Be prepared to hurt. The soreness you'll experience after exercise is a good thing. Intense work-outs disrupt our bodies' natural equilibrium by raising our temperature, and we accumulate by-products in our systems as carbohydrates combust in the absence of oxygen. (Lactic acid is probably the best known example of these by-products, but there are others too.) Once your work-out is over, your body will

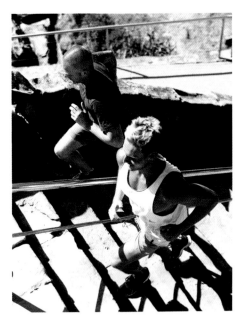

try to restore equilibrium, and this requires energy – so the harder you work out, the more you'll hurt afterwards, and the more energy you'll burn up in the repair process.

We are proponents of short, intense work-outs that target compound movements and incorporate primal elements.

An intense work-out is characterised by a significant rise in your heart rate. What you're aiming for is to get your heart pumping at 80 per cent of your maximum heart rate. Working at this intensity will lead to muscle fatigue faster than a less intense but longer session. It is therefore important to structure your work-out to allow for this. One option is to incorporate intervals: doing an exercise or a certain number of reps before taking a predetermined rest and then repeating the exercise. Another option – and one that we are a big fan of – is to work another body part (you could switch between upper and lower body) or the opposite arm or leg while you recover from the previous exercise. This approach helps create flow, increasing your body's aerobic response.

To build up your aerobic capabilities, you need to raise your heart rate to at least 60 per cent of your maximum heart rate. At 60 per cent, there are changes at the cellular level, as adaptation takes place. Peripheral changes at the vascular level start at around 70 per cent of maximum heart rate, and at 80 per cent there are changes to the heart's performance.

So, to sum up: train like the primal beast that we all are, and you'll be on your way to a stronger, fitter, healthier body. See pages 136–138 for our primal fitness plan when you're ready to get started.

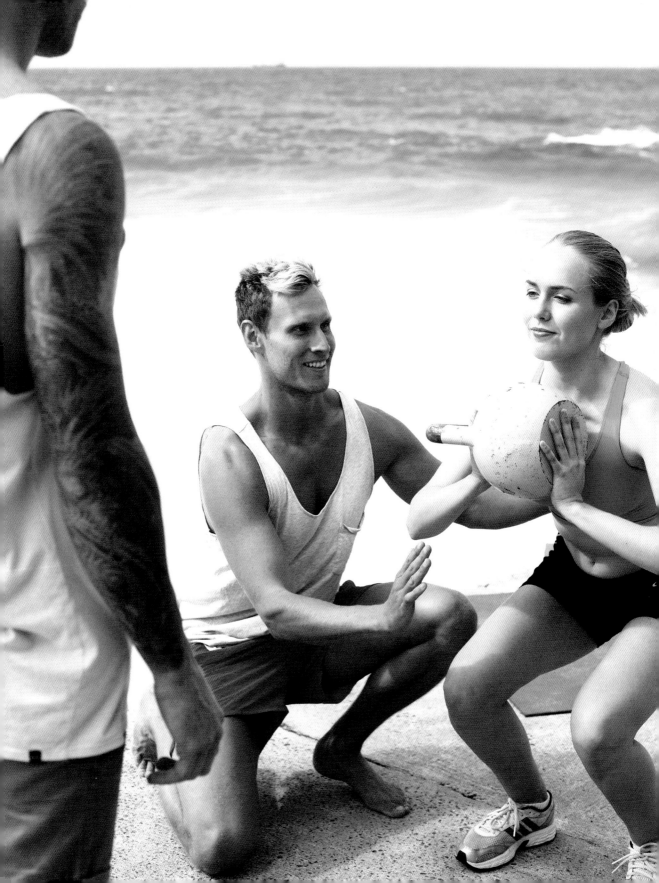

Think Right

Being equipped with the best training tools and the cleanest nutrition plan does not necessarily equal ultimate health. There is one more piece to the puzzle, and without it, your training and eating programs are at risk of failing. That missing piece is the right state of mind. You might have all the best intentions, planning to train hard and eat clean, but if you're not locked in mentally, it'll be a struggle. We believe the best way to get your mind right is through a combination of knowledge and listening to your body. Get your mind right and the rest will follow.

Learn

One obstacle when you're trying to stick to a fitness or nutrition plan is not being sure which direction to head in, or what to do next. We want to give you the knowledge you need to feel informed and confident about making healthy decisions. To do this, it's crucial to understand the principles of good nutrition and fitness.

We believe in the paleo philosophy of eating, which is currently gaining massive mainstream attention. The paleo diet is the hunter-gatherer diet and is built around foods our ancestors would have had access to. It's high in protein, veggies, fruit, nuts and seeds. Our ancestors didn't eat grains, refined sugars or dairy products, and neither should we if we want to achieve optimal health. Eating paleo is not a quick fix or a fad diet, though – it's a lifestyle. Making big changes to the way you eat can be challenging, so both your mind and body need to be plugged in and switched on if you're going to stick to it. You need to have a firm grasp of the philosophy, and of course the dos and don'ts. See pages 3–5 for more on our clean eating philosophy.

You also need to understand how your body works, how exercise affects it, and how to structure your program to reach your fitness goals. Understanding the philosophy and science behind your training program gives your work-out sessions meaning and purpose. If you understand *why* we perform squats or kettlebell swings, it will help you to persevere with them, even when you're finding them challenging. This knowledge will give you focus and centre your drive and energy. See pages 6–8 for more on our primal movement philosophy.

Listen

'Listen to your body' is a phrase that gets thrown around a great deal, but what does it actually mean? Our bodies are the incredible result of millions of years of evolution, yet in the modern world we often fail to give them the respect they deserve. We live in a fast-paced society full of distractions and noise, and we're constantly under pressure, trying to balance family and relationships with our responsibilities at work. All these factors can contribute to acute and often chronic stress. Stress affects you physically, and over long periods of time can be damaging to your health.

Our bodies evolved to deal with stressful situations in one of two ways: fight or flight. This served our ancestors well, and it's one reason they survived and passed their genes down to us. Unfortunately, our bodies still respond to stress in this way, even though we lead lives very different to those of our ancestors. The human body can't differentiate between a legitimate threat to our survival or simple stress at work, so it reacts in the same way to both. The sympathetic nervous system is activated, telling our bodies that we need an immediate source of energy. Adrenalin is pumped out; glucose is released and absorbed as fuel with the help of insulin; our heart rate goes up, and our blood pressure increases. All of this happens – and you probably haven't even left your desk. Your body responds to an unexpected email from your boss the same way it would react to a poisonous snake or a charging rhino. This is why we sometimes feel so drained at the end of the day. Our system has been in overdrive, and our stores of energy are running low.

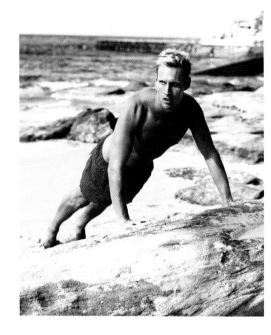

Feeling tired or run-down is your body's way of telling you to rest and recuperate. If you want to stick to your training program and see results, it's vitally important to listen to what your body is saying. Ask yourself why you are feeling tired, and where the stress is coming from. Can you avoid it or reduce it? If you're feeling exhausted, indulge yourself with a massage, an ocean swim or a social catch-up. 'Treating' yourself will pay dividends – you'll feel refreshed and relaxed, and ready to go on with your training.

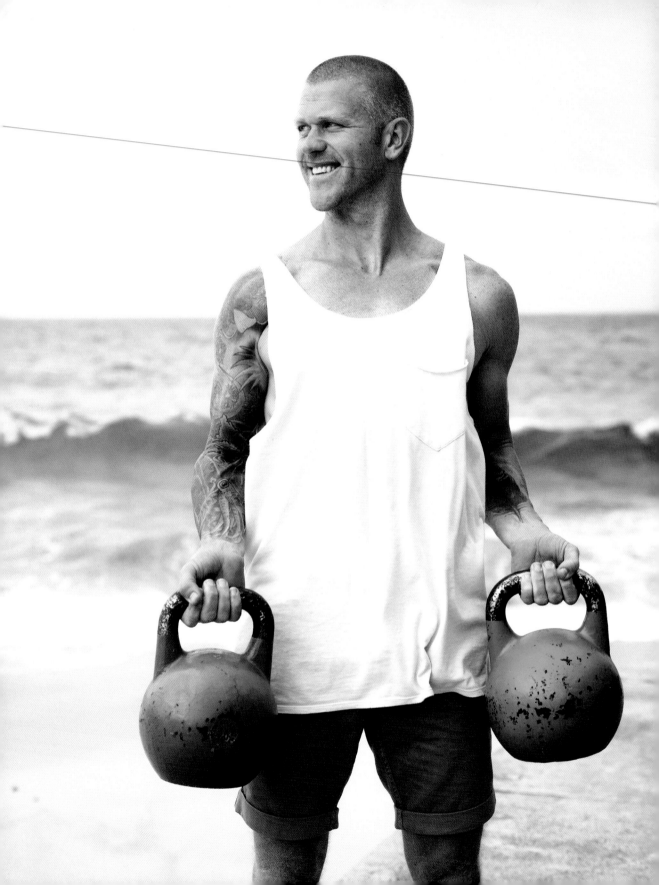

Scott's story

I know all too well what happens when we don't listen to our bodies. I used to train every day, run every day and work out without a thought for the wear and tear my body suffered. Then, about eight years ago, I ruptured three lumbar discs. When the injury first occurred I could barely walk, but still foolishly attempted to go for a run. It didn't last long. I spent most of the next six months lying on the floor. I thought my training days were pretty much gone for good. I couldn't even lift my son. For years I was in a cycle of pain and inflammation. As a personal trainer, this was far from ideal, and it affected my work. During the bad times I would get quite blue and often felt overwhelmed.

During these toughest days I had to dig deep to keep going and have faith that my injury would get better. I tried to go easy on myself and did my best not to indulge in self-pity. I'm not going to lie – things were hard – but I did stay on track with clean nutrition, even during long periods of chronic pain. The crucial point is that I tried to stay positive and focused. I searched high and low for a remedy, trying everything from invasive surgery to healing hands. That incessant search finally led me to the one specialist chiropractor who could fix me, and fixed me good. I no longer suffer from back pain and am able to train as I please. I am happy to say that lifting my son is a great deal easier and more pleasurable now.

In the end, we are the only ones who can control our actions, and it's important not to lose sight of that. Remembering this really helped me to cope with, and eventually overcome, my injury. Listen to your body – it's an incredible organism, highly sensitive yet robust. It has ways and means of communicating with you, so try to tune in. I now make it a habit to listen to my body, and I do what it tells me. When I need to rest, I rest – and the results of my training are even better now than they were before.

Recover Right

We believe rest and recovery are just as important as how you move, fuel and think about your body. Without rest, we don't repair. And without repair, we don't grow. In fact, if we don't get enough rest we risk hindering our progress, despite all our dedication to training and clean eating. Lack of rest can result in us holding onto unnecessary weight, and generally not feeling as fantastic as we possibly could. By combining good-quality sleep with the best fuel around, and adding things like yoga and meditation into your life, you will look and feel great, and you won't risk losing muscle mass.

Sleep

When we sleep, our body is given the chance to recover from the stress we've experienced during the day. This stress can be physical (in the form of strength training, for example), but it can also be the mental stress of everyday life. While we sleep we are resting and repairing our mind and body, ready for the day ahead – yet many of us don't get enough. Insufficient sleep can affect our hormone balance, leading to unwanted weight gain, mood disorders and overall lack of energy. We recommend no less than seven hours' sleep per night, but around eight to ten hours is ideal. If you adjust your lifestyle to allow for more sleep, you will see and feel the difference – we guarantee it. More sleep will make you happier, healthier, fitter, stronger and better able to deal with stress. By increasing your daily rest, you will see dramatic improvements in your mood, energy levels and overall wellbeing.

Meditate

Without getting too Bondi hipster on you, we really do want to recommend yoga and meditation. They can be an amazing reprieve from your everyday schedule. Just taking a little time out to practise mindfulness can reduce stress levels, helping you to maintain a healthy mind and to focus on what you need to get done. Exercise and good nutrition are great, but when they're combined with yoga and meditation they're even better. The outcome is a special kind of positive synergy – the yoga and meditation improve the results you see from eating and training right, and the nutrition and exercise make your yoga and meditation sessions even more rewarding. Each of these activities is more powerful and effective in combination with the others than it would be if performed separately. Take some time out for you. There is nothing more rewarding than truly looking after yourself and giving your mind and body the time they deserve.

Refuel

When you are taking time out from your fitness program to recuperate after all your hard work, make sure you fuel your body with the right stuff. Your muscles aren't actually getting stronger, or bigger, or better, in the gym. You are tearing them apart and breaking them down. It is only by resting and refuelling after exercise that we become stronger, faster and more toned. Don't think that because you have trained you can pig out on a high-calorie meal, however – your body needs healthy carbs and protein. Smart choices and optimal nutrition will lead to long-term results you will be happy with. Remember, the satisfaction of success far outweighs the brief moment of temptation. The recipes we've included in this book will fuel your body and delight your tastebuds as well!

Losing muscle v. losing fat

It's so important not to overdo it! When we overtrain to try to fast-track results, we usually end up in the catabolic zone. This is basically when we have no carbs to burn as energy, so we burn our muscle mass away. Muscle tissue is readily used as energy when our other sources of energy are depleted; this can happen so easily if we don't give our bodies enough time to rest. Muscle burns more calories than fat, so maintaining lean muscle mass throughout your life keeps fat loss from slowing. Building muscle mass might actually *add* weight as it replaces less dense fatty tissue, so don't freak out if one day you're slightly heavier, even though you feel better than ever. It just means you are gaining lean muscle mass, and because exercise depends on muscle strength, those who maintain muscle mass have greater exercise tolerance and endurance. A continued program of exercise and healthy eating leads to lasting results. If you avoid quick fixes you will look and feel amazing.

Stay Motivated

Staying on track with your new healthy lifestyle isn't always easy. We've made our guide to health and fitness simple, so you can stick to it without trouble, but even the most disciplined among us occasionally loses our grip. So how can you stay motivated?

Evaluate

First, evaluate your current routine and habits. Are you happy with the life you're living now, or is there a better version of yourself hidden somewhere inside? What could you do differently? Think about fitness and nutrition as you ask yourself these questions:

Are you happy with your training? Is it producing the best results? Are you doing enough, or could you squeeze in a little more?

For a week, analyse the feeling you get once you've eaten. How do you feel five to ten minutes after breakfast, lunch or dinner? Your body will tell you if you're not eating right. Look out for signs like lethargy, sleepiness and bloating. Make a list of the foods that make you feel sluggish and then get rid of them. Stock your fridge and cupboard with nutrient-dense fresh food that will fill you up with life and energy.

Set goals

The next step is to set goals based on where you are currently and where you want to be. The key to setting successful goals is to make them realistic and achievable – anything else will only lead to disappointment. The goals can be simple – for example, 'I'm going to eat fresh fish three times this week', or 'I'm going to train an extra day this week'.

Set short- and long-term goals. Short-term goals can be daily or weekly, and long-term goals should be monthly or quarterly. Write them down and keep them somewhere where you'll see them – in your wallet, for example, or at your desk. This acts as a constant reminder.

It can help to confide your goals to a friend, partner or colleague – someone who can support you but who will also hold you to account. As personal trainers, we believe that setting goals with clients is the best way to start a program – that way you both have clearly defined roles and responsibilities.

If you do happen to miss your goal, don't see it as a failure. Use it as a motivator to help you hit the next one. Remember, health and fitness is a lifestyle – there's always room for improvement and never a reason to drop off. Our philosophy is not about quick fixes or fads – it's about education, clean nutrition and effective training over the long term, to help you be the best you can be every day.

Your first goal is to finish reading this book and then make a start.

Plan

The next step is planning. Once you have set your goals you need a concrete plan that will help you reach them. Don't worry – it need not involve charts, graphs and hours of your time. It can be as simple as grabbing your groceries at the start of the week so you can cook healthy meals when you get home at night, or taking your work-out gear to work with you.

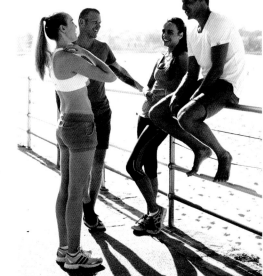

We can't stress enough the benefits of having a fridge stocked full of clean food. For starters, it eliminates the risk of grabbing something unhealthy just because it's convenient. Plan ahead and your health will thank you.

Reassess

Health and fitness is a continuum – it has no end point – so don't be too disappointed with yourself if you drop the ball once in a while. There's always time to reflect and reassess, and it's vital that you do so. The key to staying on track is being happy with your fitness routine and your nutrition. If one or both are 'hard work', there's a strong chance you won't stick to them. The wonderful thing about our philosophy and our program is that they offer freedom and choice – so if you're not happy with something, just change it. There's never any need to feel bored or stale.

Good luck – and remember that health and fitness are a lifestyle choice, not a quick fix!

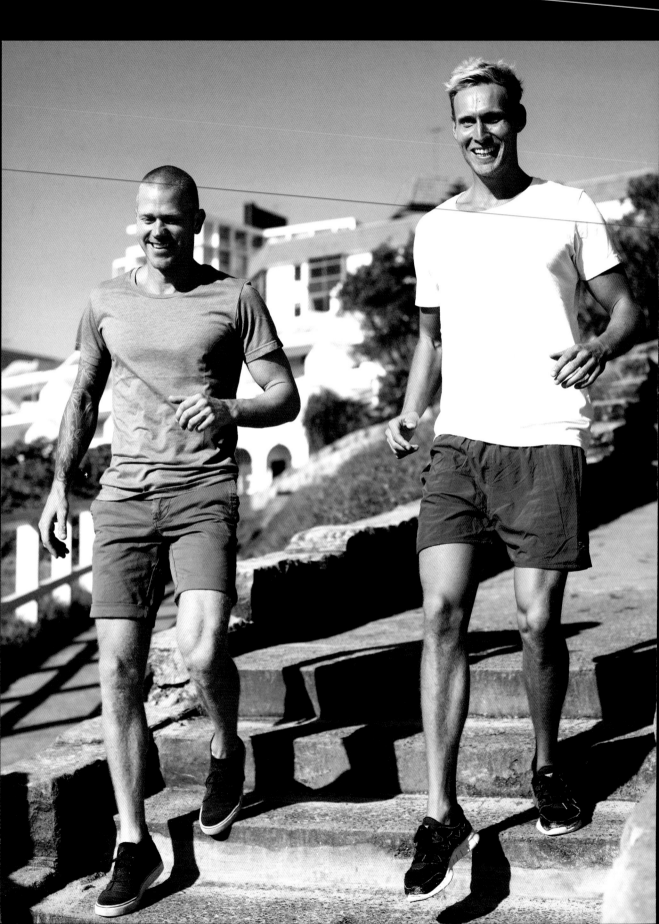

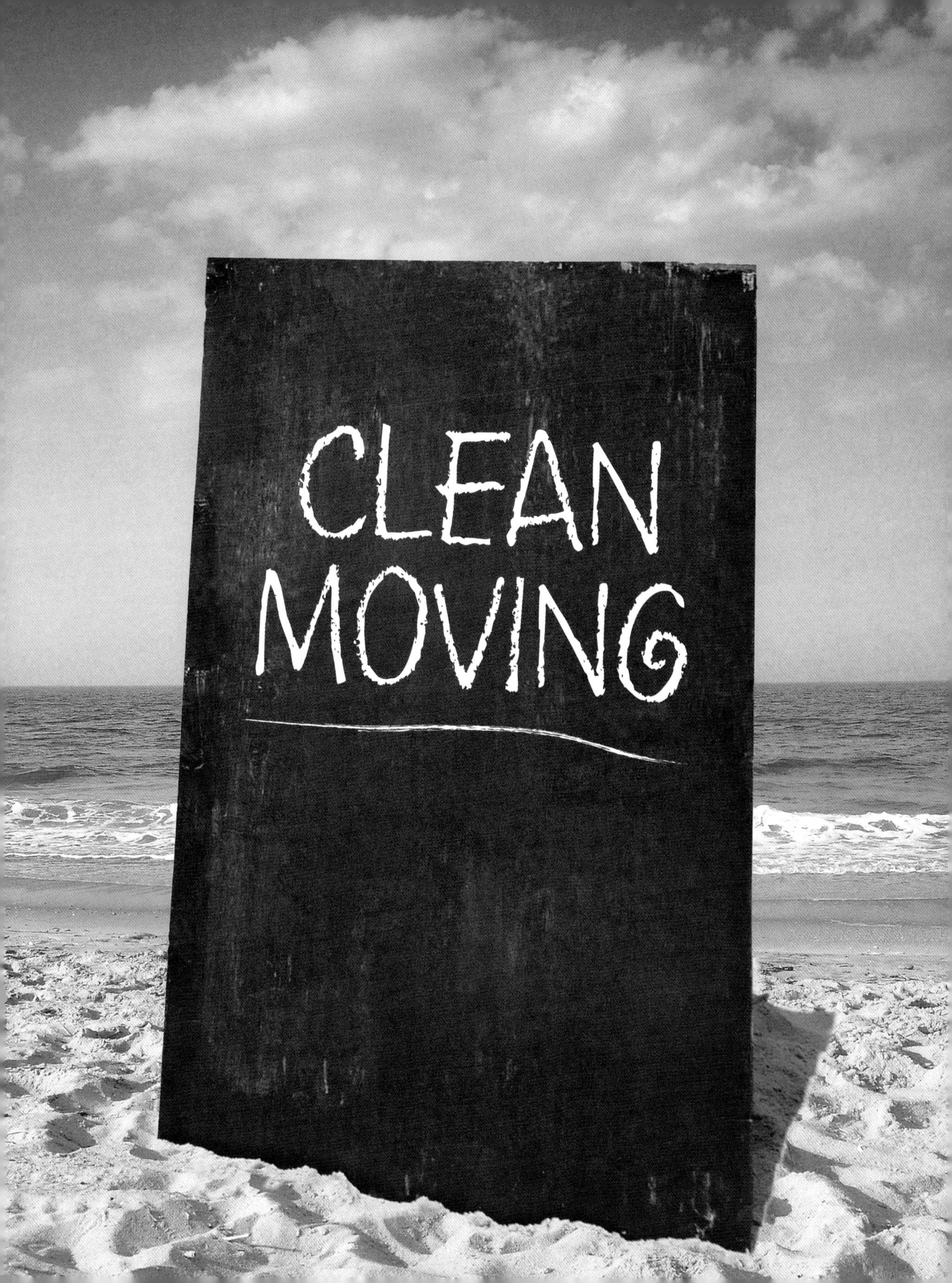
CLEAN
MOVING

Fitness Philosophy

Exercise has never been more important. We live in a world of distractions, convenience food and quick-fix attitudes. For optimal health it's vital to move your body in the way it is designed to move, but exercise is often neglected or, at the other extreme, abused. Too little exercise is bad for us, but ill-prescribed exercise is also detrimental to our health.

Exercise should be something you enjoy. It should be primal and it should be functional and practical.

It's no secret that regular exercise works wonders for your body and mind. The physiological benefits are almost too many to mention, but here are just a few reasons to train.

Regular exercise ...

- builds strong muscles, tendons, ligaments and bones

- retards ageing

- promotes a positive outlook and releases hormones such as endorphins and serotonin that make you feel happy

- improves the distribution of oxygen to your muscles, allowing you to work harder for longer

- stimulates the nervous system

- increases your metabolism.

Training need not be time-consuming or expensive – we like to make it accessible, simple and quick. There's no better way to kickstart your day than by giving all the major muscle groups a work-out that leaves you feeling strong, empowered, confident and invigorated.

To understand our fitness philosophy, it's necessary to understand a little bit about us. Despite very different upbringings and backgrounds, we share one thing, which is that we strive to be the best version of ourselves that we can possibly be. For us, that comes from training and good, clean nutrition. We have had a long interest in training and have tried various sports, disciplines and even the odd fad, but we always come back to functional training. Functional training mimics the sorts of movements you use in everyday life – lifting, pulling, pushing and so on – the primal movements our bodies were designed to make. Functional training is almost the default for us – in our opinion, it's the most effective way to train.

We prescribe exercise and training for our clients daily, and have done for years. Through experience, knowledge and learning we've discovered the most effective way to move our bodies. This training is best done in unison with a clean, nutrient-rich diet. One supports the other and they work in synergy for optimal health.

It's important to note here, before we go on, that you should always seek medical clearance before starting a new training regimen if you haven't trained regularly in a while or have concerns about your health. Our exercises are designed for people cleared 'fit' for strenuous exercise. Head to your GP if you're unsure.

We believe the best way to train is to constantly test yourself, and test yourself in different ways. As we know, the human body is an amazing piece of engineering, and readily adapts in response to stress. For example, if you decide to run five kilometres one day after years of not running, you would probably find it uncomfortable or even impossible, but if you try to run that distance again it will be a little easier. If you continue over time, your body will adapt and eventually you'll be running five kilometres with no trouble. This phenomenon is known as overcompensation. Overcompensation occurs when the body is placed under stress and reacts by adapting, so that when the body is exposed to the same stress again it will be easier to deal with. This is what makes it possible to get fitter. It's therefore imperative to stress the body not only frequently but also in different ways, to ensure constant growth and to avoid staleness.

We believe in complete or full-body fitness – training every part of the body using various modes of exercise (such as weights, calisthenics or boxing) to develop the different facets of fitness (strength, speed, power and endurance). You can vary your exercise to focus on a specific facet by modifying your reps, sets, duration, speed or load. Remember, your body will only become conditioned to what you expose it to. So vary the mode of exercise and the facet you focus on to ensure well-rounded fitness.

If you don't train hard, there will be no need for the body to adapt and grow. We propose that you work as hard as you can for your allotted work-out time to put your body under the greatest stress you can. This training style will promote the most rapid development in fitness levels. But how long should you train for? It's long been considered that we need to train the body for up to thirty minutes for significant changes to take place. We advocate a much shorter time frame. Along with many other fitness experts, coaches and physiologists, we believe that you can do an extremely efficient and effective training session in a fraction of that time. Take the work of Izumi Tabata, for instance – a Japanese physiologist who devised a four-minute training protocol that improves anaerobic and aerobic function. This protocol relies on you working as hard as you can for just four minutes, broken down into eight bursts of intense work lasting twenty seconds, each followed by ten seconds of rest. This form of training achieves results – and is perfectly tailored for us time-poor folks.

Tabata's training protocol relies on you working as hard as *you* can – it's not about comparing yourself to others – and this is part of our approach too. We've been running boot camps and corporate groups for years, and we always stress the importance of the individual and ask participants not to compare themselves to others. If you are working hard, that's all that can be asked of you.

We live in sophisticated societies, but strip that away and you're left with primal beings with primal needs and instincts. Our training style is based on this belief. Humans are designed to run, jump, pull, push, lift, drag and climb. We are naturally capable of all these actions, but we don't always make good use of them in the modern world. Training should foster our natural abilities and develop them, so that we can perform them all equally well and are not dominant in one. Being strong in one area while we are weak in others can lead to imbalances and potential overuse injuries. Our ancestors needed full-body fitness to survive. We just need to translate that into our modern world.

To sum up, our underlying ethos is: Just as nature intended! We don't believe in quick fixes or short cuts with training, so no non-natural supplements. To reach your goals, all you need is clean nutrition – food in its most natural state, which is nutrient-dense – and regular training. Keep your mind and body strong and you can achieve optimal health. That's what clean living is all about.

The Exercises Explained

The exercises in this section will provide you with the tools for a strong body. We'll describe the basic form of each exercise and then tell you how to modify it to suit your individual needs. Some terms that will help you understand these exercises are listed below.

Adaptation

When we train, we are essentially 'stressing' the body. In the days following a training session the body will repair the damage done, and, if you continue to exercise, it will actually improve, leaving you a little stronger and fitter than before. This phenomenon is called overcompensation. The adaptations your body makes will reflect the type of training you do, as well as the level of intensity. The adaptation phase lasts up to 72 hours, after which time any improvements gained are lost, so the adage 'use it or lose it' is very much true.

Calisthenics

Calisthenics is a form of training that uses body weight for resistance, rather than equipment. The scope of movements is vast, from simple movements such as jumping, bending and stretching, to more complex movements. Calisthenics is used to build strength, flexibility and cardiovascular fitness.

Core Muscles

There is a degree of ambiguity about the definition of 'core muscles'. Your absolute core muscles are those deep-lying muscles, the primary function of which is to stabilise your spine and safeguard you from excessive spinal movements that could cause injury. However, the term is also used to describe the muscles that drive functional movement – your hamstrings, gluteals and abdominals.

Functional Training

'Functional training' is a style of training that utilises full-body exercises (i.e. upper and lower body at the same time). These exercises involve compound movements – that is, movements that use more than one joint – and rely heavily on the core muscles. Functional training has practical benefits and should improve your everyday movements and physical tasks, such as lifting or climbing stairs. Functional training includes, but is not limited to, pushing, pulling, lifting, dragging and climbing.

High Plank

Many exercises start with the 'high plank' position. Start by lying prone (face down), resting on your hands and toes. Your hands should be under your shoulders, with the inside of your elbow facing forward and your elbow locked. Your feet should be positioned shoulder-width apart. Curl your toes under for comfort. Your glutes and abs should be switched on to ensure stability. (See page 35 for more info.)

Lactic Acid

Our body strives for an equilibrium known as 'homeostasis' – the state of wellbeing we enjoy when our systems are in balance. Exercise stresses the body, disrupting this equilibrium, and can lead to chemical by-products accumulating in our systems. Lactic acid is one of these by-products. It accumulates in the blood and other body tissues, lowering the body's natural pH, which is why we feel yuck when we train hard. Our ability to tolerate lactic acid and other by-products of intense exercise increases as we get fitter and stronger – so don't let that yucky feeling deter you!

Muscle Soreness

Your training should generate some degree of muscle soreness. If it doesn't, it's probably necessary to change or evolve your regime. Muscle soreness or DOMS (delayed onset of muscle soreness) peaks 48 hours after exercising and may last up to 72 hours. Even when your muscles are very sore, the best option is to keep using them, rather than resting – movement and contraction promote blood flow and repair.

Neutral Spine

A typical spine exhibits four natural curves: the cervical, the thoracic, the lumbar and the sacral curve (or, in plain English, the neck, the upper back, the lower back and the pelvic curve). When the body is properly aligned, all four curves should be present and in balance. This is known as 'neutral spine' (or 'good posture'). When we move, those four curves are often compromised, but our core muscles work to stabilise us, keeping the curves in balance. Excessive deviation from neutral spine can inhibit our core muscles and expose us to potential injury. It is therefore crucial to condition your core muscles, and core training should be an integral part of your routine.

Plyometrics

Our muscles are like elastic: once they are stretched, they are primed for contraction. When this contraction occurs at high speed, it can generate explosive power. Plyometrics is an advanced form of training that harnesses this power to build speed and strength. Plyometrics exercises typically lengthen the target muscle and then use the following contraction to power the next movement – for example, in a series of jumps or bounds. It requires a great deal of energy not only to perform the 'hard' phase but also to control and decelerate the movement.

Range of Motion

Each joint has tendons attached, which pull on it to produce movement, and ligaments, which hold it in place. Each joint has a particular 'range of motion', determining how freely and how far the joint can move, and in which directions. This differs from person to person. When you exercise, we recommend that you work each joint through its full range of motion, if possible, as this will promote strength throughout the entire range and safeguard you from injury.

Supine + Prone

'Supine' means lying on your back, face up. You are supine as you prepare to do a crunch. 'Prone' is the opposite. You are prone when you are in the plank position.

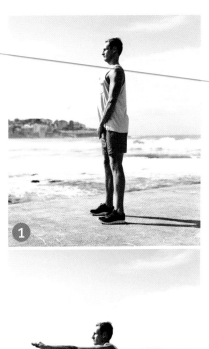

The Squat

This is a foundation exercise that primarily activates the glutes, quads and core. Squats are extremely effective and can be used for a vast range of training goals, from toning to power lifting.

Mechanics

Stand with your feet shoulder-width apart and slightly angled out.

Bending at the hip, lower yourself into the squat position. As you descend, use your arms as a counterbalance to keep you stable. Stick your bum out as your torso leans forwards, and maintain a straight back. Straight – not vertical!

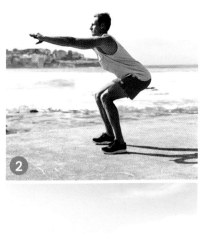

Bend your knees until you are in a full squat position. The angle of your back should be the same as the angle between your knee and your ankle. Use a mirror to check that you have got it right.

Go as deep as you can while still maintaining the correct angle. Don't be afraid to stick your bum out! Ensure your weight is placed over your heels and not your toes. You should be able to wiggle your toes at the bottom of the squat.

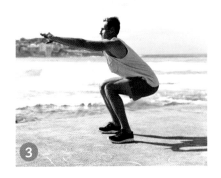

Return to the starting position by driving your weight through your heels to give your glutes a real work-out.

Variations

Easier ... Place a stool or chair behind you. From your start position, lower your bum until it gently taps the seat behind you, then return to the start position. Over time, use a lower gauge, until you can perform a squat unassisted.

Harder ... Try a squat jump. Squat jumps will develop muscle tone quicker and improve your aerobic fitness – double tick! From the bottom of the squat, drive down through your heels and at the same time drive the arms to help you lift off the ground. Land on your forefoot and roll onto your heels before descending again for another rep. Before attempting continuous reps, first try one rep and pause in the start position. Once you have control and feel stable, try continuous reps for maximum results.

Even harder ... Grab a weight, such as a dumbbell, kettlebell or bag of sand, and keep it close to your chest as your perform your squat. Keep your weight over your heels, and ensure your back stays straight.

> **TIP:** The wider your stance, the harder your inner thighs will have to work. As you increase the distance between your feet, angle them out a little more.

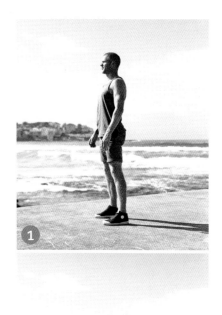

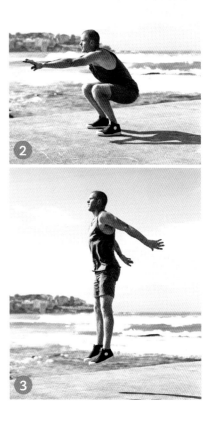

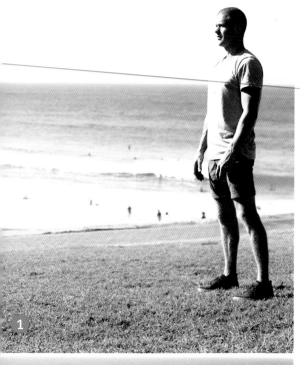

The Elephant Walk

This is a core-driven exercise that also works the shoulders, chest and hamstrings. Doing continuous reps will give you an aerobic work-out.

Mechanics

Stand with your feet slightly wider than shoulder-width apart and slightly angled out.

Bend at the hips and allow your hands to touch the floor close to your feet. Keep your knees straight, if you can, or bend them slightly if you need to.

Keeping your hips as stable as possible, walk your hands out away from your feet until you feel your abs kick in. Your hands and feet should be as far apart as they can be without compromising your neutral spine.

Hold this position for two to five seconds before walking your hands back to your feet, then return to a standing position.

Variations

Harder ... Do the standard elephant walk described above, but start with your feet a little closer together. Maintain control of your core and try not to rock your hips.

Even harder ... Once your hands are under your shoulders, do a push-up, then walk your hands back to their starting position, at your feet.

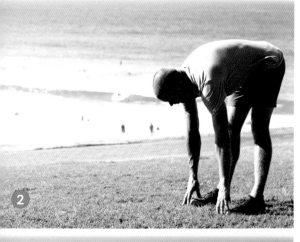

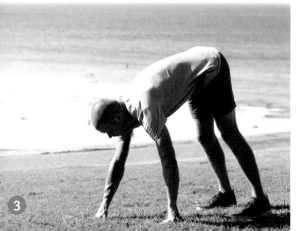

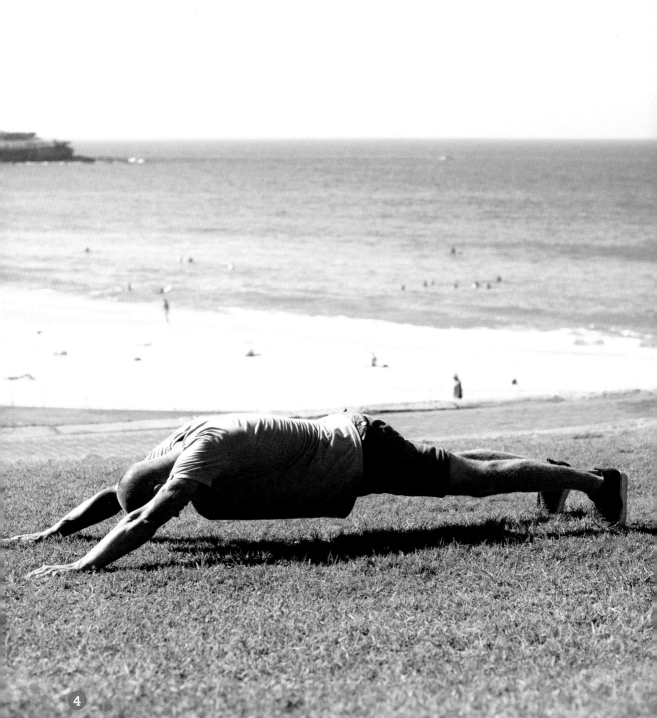

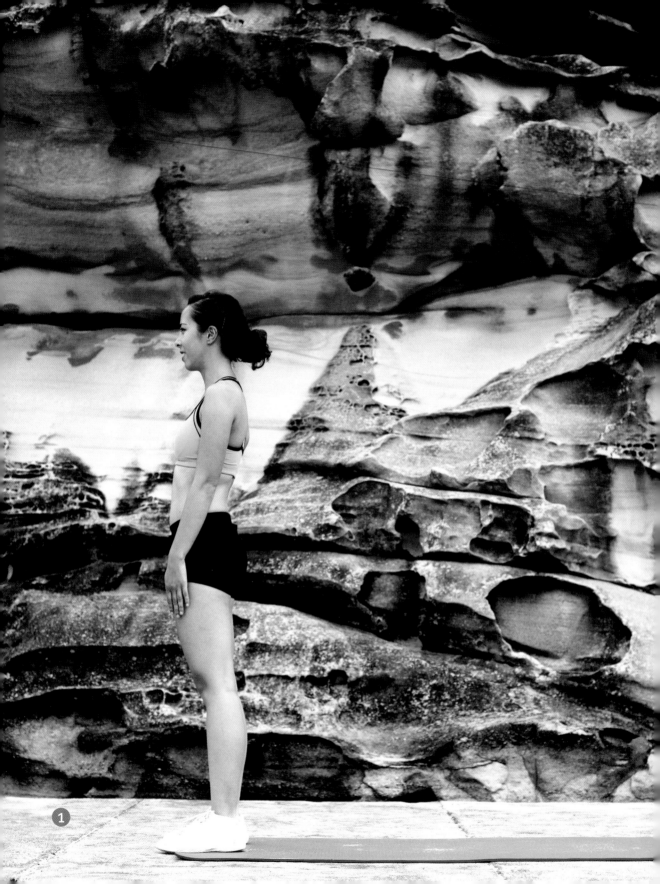

The Roll-back with Kick-up

This exercise recruits all the major muscle groups. There's very little of you not working during this exercise – it's great for abs, core and legs. It requires coordination, control, agility and strength. Once you combine all those elements and do a few reps, it becomes a demanding aerobic work-out. It's a little tricky to master, and you won't get it on your first go, but stick with it and you'll notice the difference.

Mechanics

Stand with your mat behind you.

Bend at the hips and knees, as if to perform a squat (see instructions on page 26). Sink low, until you can place your hands on the floor just behind you.

Lean your weight over your heels until you rock backwards, then roll along your spine until your weight is over your shoulders.

From this position, kick up, driving your feet vertically into the air.

Keeping up both your speed and momentum, reverse the kick-up and roll-back actions until you are back on your feet in the start position.

Variation

Easier ... Do the roll-back component of the exercise, but don't kick up. Instead, roll onto your shoulders, getting good range of motion through the spine before driving forwards again, back to your feet and to the start position.

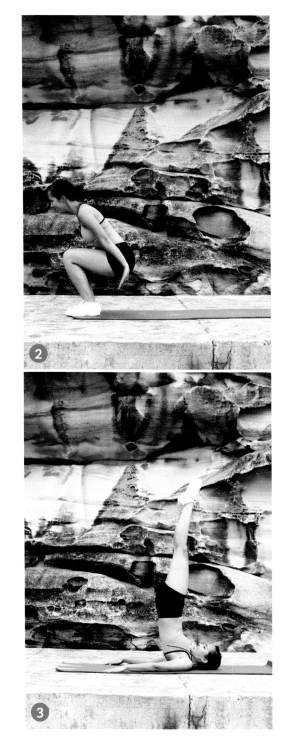

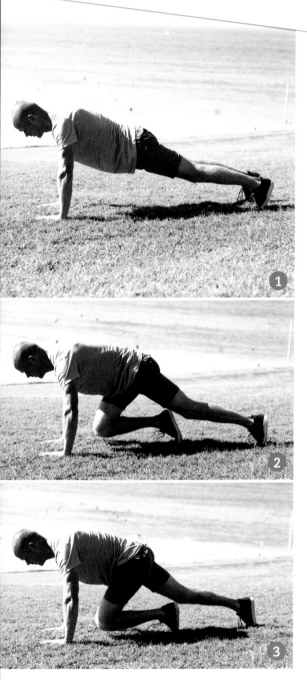

The Mountain Climber

This is a dynamic exercise that really taxes the midsection and is incredibly aerobic. It uses the core, abdominals and shoulders.

Mechanics

Lie face down with your hands underneath your shoulders and your hips flat – similar to a push-up position with your feet together. For comfort, turn your fingers out to the side and push the inside of your elbow joints forwards.

Lock your elbows and drive one knee high up into your chest, then return your leg to the start position.

Repeat using the opposite leg. For the best results, continuously alternate legs, almost bouncing from one leg to the other.

Variations

Harder ... Rather than driving the knee directly towards your chest, aim it towards your opposite wrist. Rotating the hip and torso like this targets the obliques like crazy.

Even harder ... Increase the range of motion by bringing your leg across your body until your foot is in line with your hands. Your little toe should be closest to the ground. This version is not for the faint-hearted. We call these ones windscreen wipers.

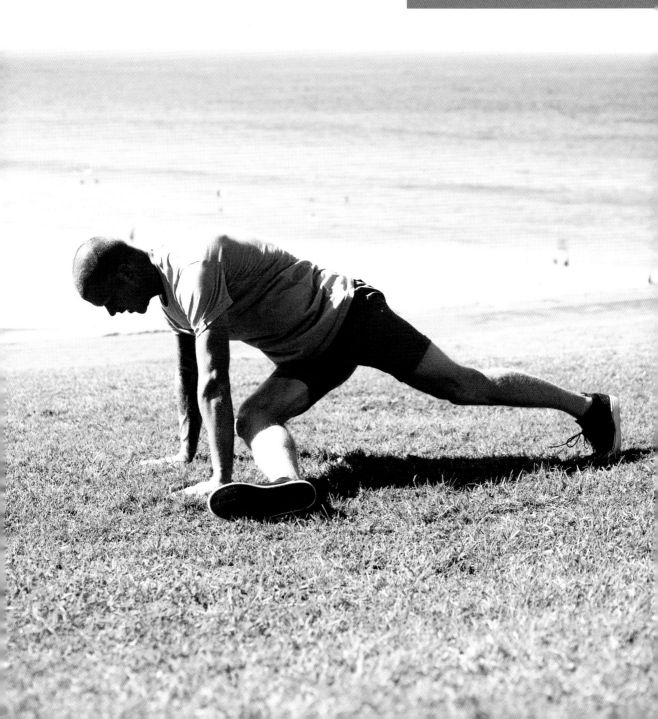

TIP: To give your core a really good work-out, keep your hips nice and flat.

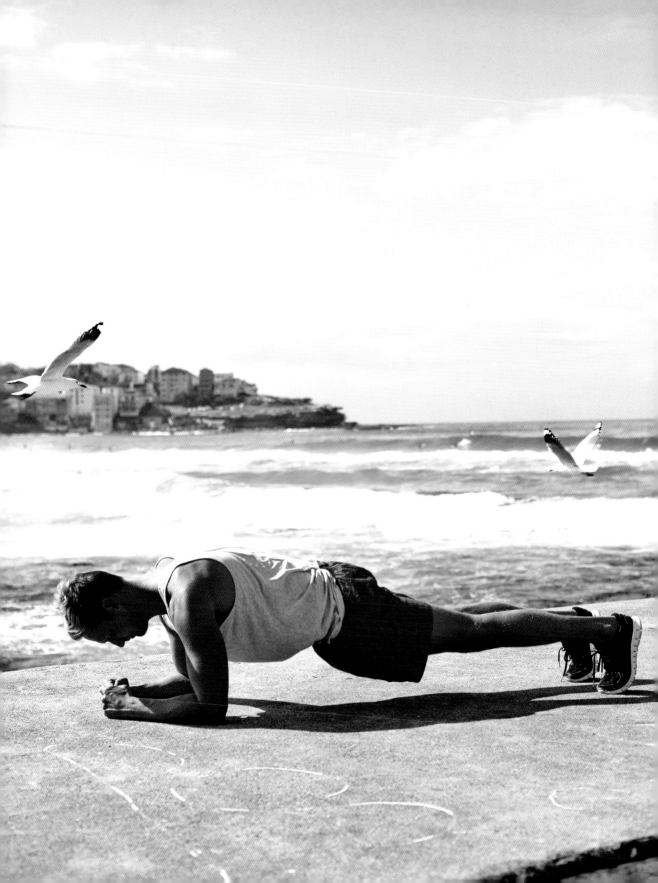

The Plank

This is a tried-and-tested exercise and a great way to build core strength. To do the plank you lie face down, supported by your feet and forearms. Your midsection has no support, so your core muscles have to work hard. It's a static exercise, but you can easily increase the complexity and intensity of the work-out by removing points of contact.

Mechanics

Lie face down, resting on your forearms and toes. Your elbows should be beneath your shoulders, and your feet should be close together, or even touching. Curl your toes under for comfort.

Keep your spine neutral and your hips in line with your shoulders. Check in a mirror – if your hips are too high, you won't be using the target muscles.

Hold this position for as long as you can, but leave a little in the tank so you can come down and rest on your knees with control.

Variations

Easier ... A plank is all about stressing your midsection by placing your points of contact far away from each other. This can be achieved by resting on your knees rather than your feet. The all-important thing is to ensure your spine is neutral. Hold the position for as long as you can, but leave a little in reserve so you can sink into the rest position with control.

Harder ... A classic plank has four points of contact – two forearms and two feet. Removing one or two points of contact very quickly makes the exercise more intense. The key is to keep your hips square and your spine neutral. Our advice is to move your feet a little further apart before removing a point of contact. Try wrapping one arm around your torso, as if you're giving yourself a hug. Hold this position before alternating arms. Alternatively, you can lift one leg. Keeping the leg straight, lift your foot about three to five centimetres off the ground, hold and then swap.

TIP: When you're doing the plank, your large 'global' muscles (abdominals and obliques) tend to take over from your stabilising core muscles. To stop this happening, follow these tips:

1. Breathe steadily.

2. Draw in your abdomen just above your pubic bone.

3. Contract your pelvic floor (imagine you're peeing, and stopping your flow midstream).

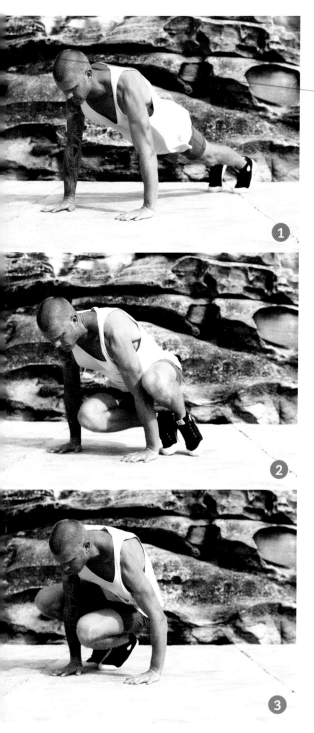

The Thruster

This is a dynamic strength- and core-based exercise that will get your heart pumping, rip your midsection and work your shoulders.

Mechanics

Lie face down in a high plank (resting on your hands rather than your forearms). Make sure your spine is neutral and your hands are under your shoulders.

Bring both your knees in towards your chest. Allow your hips to rise towards the ceiling as you bring your knees in – if you keep them flat, you'll be using your hip flexors instead of the target muscles, and you don't want that. Your spine should curve as you tuck yourself into a ball.

Return to the start position and repeat. Keep the tempo up to make the most of this aerobic exercise.

Variations

Easier ... Adjust the tempo and slow things down a little. Hold the start position for five seconds, do one thrust, then return to the start position and hold again for another five seconds before the next rep.

Harder ... Work the obliques as well as your abs – instead of bringing your knees to your chest when you thrust, bring them either side of your elbow. Your left knee should be on the inside of your right elbow and your right knee on the outside – and vice versa for the left elbow. (See illustrated examples to left.)

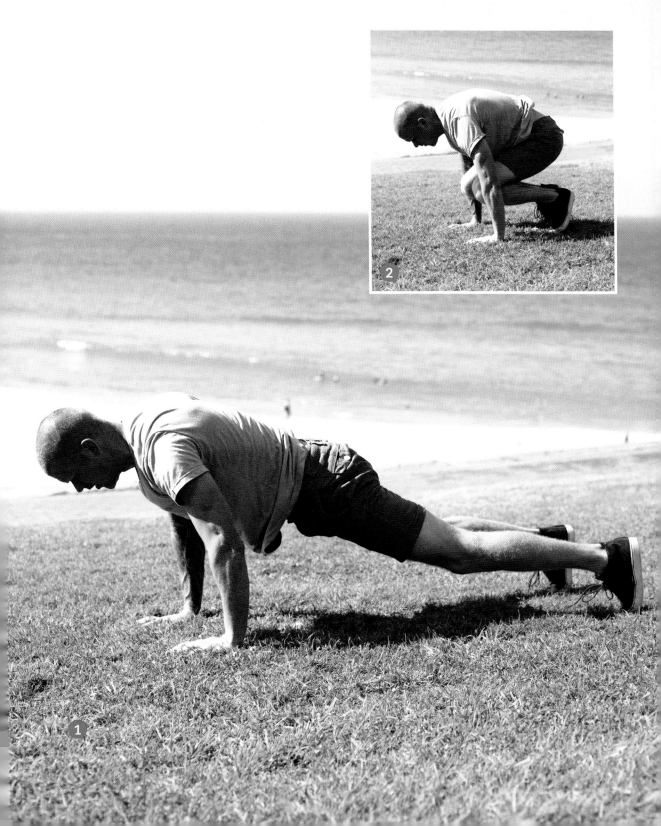

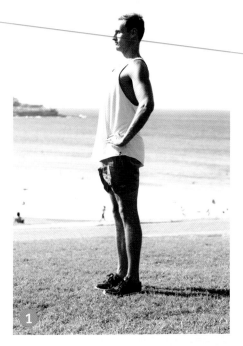

The Reverse Lunge

The reverse lunge is an absolute stalwart in the exercise world. It has been around for a long time, and it's here to stay – for a very good reason. It recruits the glutes more effectively than a front lunge, and more than deserves its inclusion in our list.

Mechanics

Stand with your feet close together. Take a long stride back with your left leg, and finish on your toes. Your toes should be tucked under and your back leg more or less straight.

Drop your back knee straight down towards the ground and allow it to flirt with the floor. The lower it goes, the harder you'll be working your glute.

Once your back knee is down as low as it can go, your hip and front knee joint should form a right angle. Use a mirror to check. If the angle is less than 90 degrees, you need to take a longer backwards stride.

Come back to your start position by driving through your right heel. Repeat using the opposite leg.

Variation

Harder ... Increase the intensity by adding weight. Do the reverse lunge holding dumbbells, kettlebells or a barbell. Pay attention to your form and ensure you drive through your front heel to get maximum benefit.

The Split Lunge

Just like its cousin the reverse lunge, the more dynamic split lunge is an absolute must for strength and cardio training. This exercise relies on strength, speed and coordination. The split lunge is great for growing and toning muscle, as well as aerobic training, but it will really make you hurt!

Mechanics

Stand with your feet close together and bounce into a split foot position. Your left foot should step forwards and your right foot should step back.

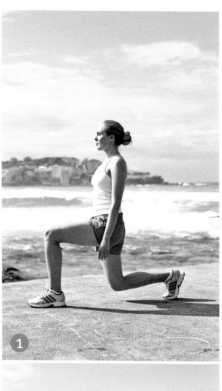

Drop the back knee and allow it to flirt with the ground. You should be able to do this without overloading your front knee. If you can't, move your feet further apart. Once your back knee is down, your hip and front knee joint should form a right angle. Use a mirror to check. Your front knee should not travel past your toes as you lunge.

Once your knee has touched the ground, jump straight through to the alternate side.

As you move, keep your shoulders pinned back and your back straight – the drive should all come via the legs. Use your arms for momentum and balance.

Allow the opposite back knee to flirt with the ground and then repeat.

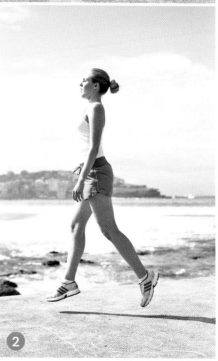

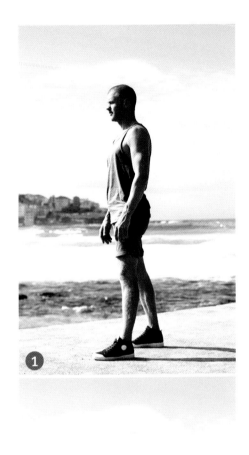

The Box Lunge

This exercise can be hard to master but is well worth it. It rotates your torso, working your midsection and obliques. It's also a great exercise for the lateral hip muscles. It requires strength, coordination and flexibility, but if flexibility isn't your strong suit, just adjust your initial foot position slightly.

Mechanics

Stand with your left foot forwards and your right slightly behind. The toes of your right foot should be in line with your left heel, a foot length apart.

Facing forwards, with your shoulders pinned back, bend at the hips and knees and lower yourself towards the ground.

Place your right hand in the space between your left heel and your right toe. The first time you try this you'll be shaky, but don't let it put you off. You'll soon adjust and the shaking will stop. Gently tap the floor, or just get as close to it as you can, then return to the start position and repeat.

Variation

Harder ... Increase the intensity by placing a medicine ball or kettlebell on your shoulder. When your right foot is forwards, hold the weight on your right side. When your left foot is forwards, hold it on your left. Before you increase the weight, check your posture. Remember: form first, then intensity.

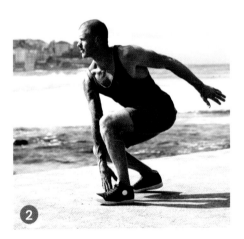

The Sprawl

The sprawl is seen in wrestling, jujitsu and mixed martial arts. When used in these sports it's a way of counteracting your opponent's offensive moves, but it's also a popular training exercise. The sprawl is particularly demanding, forcing you to work hard no matter what condition you're in.

Mechanics

Stand with your feet shoulder-width apart, then bend your hips and knees until your hands reach the floor.

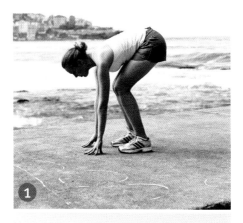

Jump back with both feet into a high plank position, ensuring your hips are in line with your shoulders, then immediately jump forwards, bringing your feet back between your hands. (This movement is similar to a thruster – see instructions on page 36.) Make sure your core muscles are switched on so that your hips don't dip, thereby putting excessive pressure on your lumbar spine.

Return to a standing position and repeat.

Variation

Harder … Throw in a push-up! Once you're in the high plank position, drop down into a push-up on your knees or your feet before bringing your feet back between your hands and returning to a standing position.

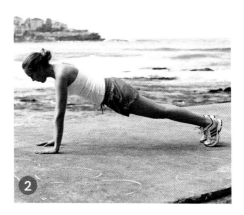

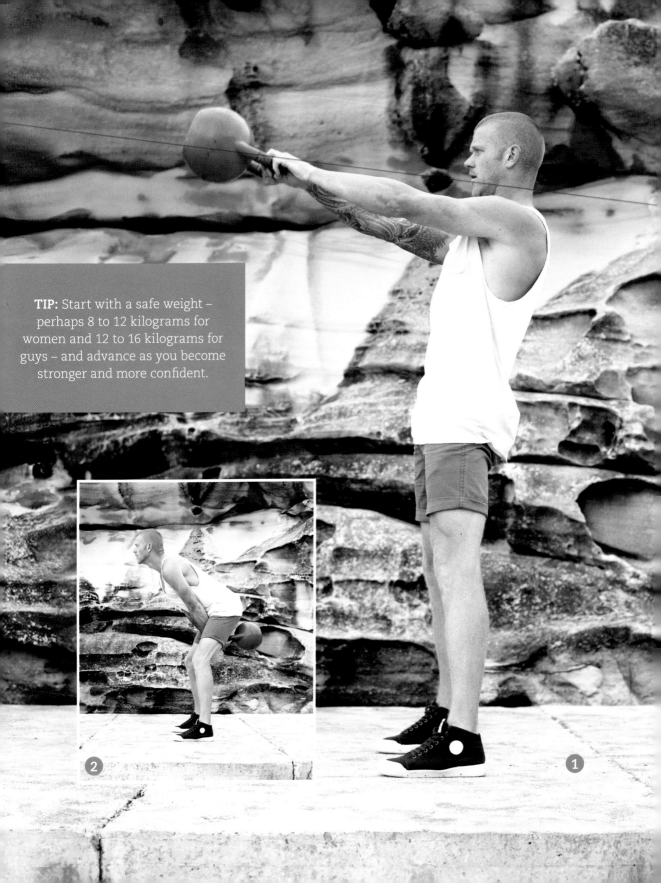

TIP: Start with a safe weight – perhaps 8 to 12 kilograms for women and 12 to 16 kilograms for guys – and advance as you become stronger and more confident.

The Kettlebell Swing

A kettlebell is a compact weight, originally developed in Russia and long used by Russian gymnasts and the military for training. The swing is considered the cornerstone exercise of kettlebell training and has been widely adopted by mainstream fitness practitioners. The kettlebell swing is a hip-dominant exercise and fantastic for developing strength, endurance and fitness. The swing is essentially a dynamic deadlift.

Mechanics

Place the kettlebell on the floor just in front of you, then stand with your feet shoulder-width apart and facing forwards.

Grip the kettlebell loosely in the fingers rather than the palm of the hand. Drag it towards you and lift it from the hips with a straight back.

'Break' your hip or punch your bum out behind you and bend your knees a little. Resist the temptation to drop into a squat, as this will recruit different muscles and not the ones you are targeting. Ensure your shoulders are pinned back and your back is straight.

Drive your hips forward into full extension and swing the kettlebell out in front of you. The hip drive will generate the power you need. Allow the handle to pivot in your fingers as you swing. Aim to get the weight up to around shoulder height. The movement must be fast and explosive. If it is too slow, you will feel discomfort in your shoulders and your lower back.

The bell of the weight should be furthest away from you at the end of the movement. As it swings back, decelerate the weight to maintain control. Break the hip again as your upper body comes forwards. Keep the elbows soft throughout the movement.

The kettlebell should swing high between your legs. If it's swinging between your knees, you're bending too much at the knees or your back is too round.

Variation

Harder … Try doing this exercise using just one hand. Once you've mastered the single-hand swing, you can alternate every rep by swapping hands at the top of the movement, when the weight is at shoulder height.

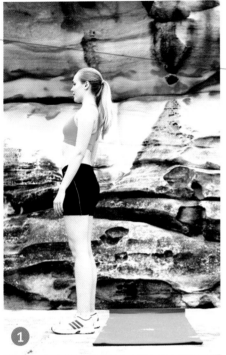

The Kneel to Standing

A simple but very effective exercise. Don't be fooled by its simplicity – as the reps build up, this exercise can start to seem incredibly demanding.

Mechanics

Stand with your feet shoulder-width apart and your mat behind you.

Take a long stride back with your left leg, over the mat, and finish on your toes. Your toes should be tucked under.

Drop your back knee straight down until it is resting on the mat. Bring your right leg to rest alongside your left.

Bend your right hip and bring your knee up so that your left foot is now on the floor in front of the mat. Your left hip and knee joint should form right angles. Use a mirror to check.

Drive down into your left heel as you come to a standing position with both feet together.

Repeat, alternating your legs to work both glutes. Ensure the movement is driven from your glutes by minimising movement from the upper body. Aim to be as stable as you can throughout the upper body.

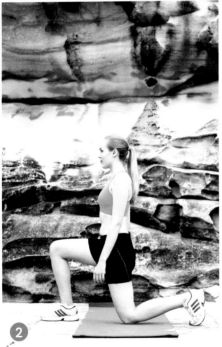

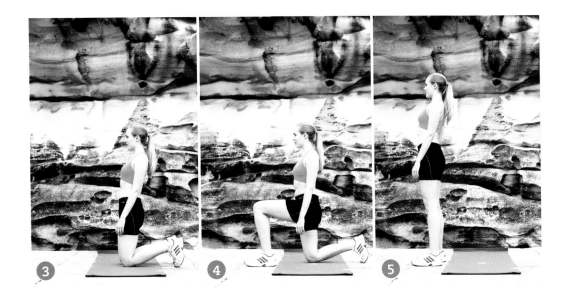

Variation

Harder ... Add weight to increase intensity. Do this exercise holding a medicine ball, dumbbell or kettlebell close to your body. Focus on form, as the additional weight will throw you off balance. Try to maintain control throughout the entire movement.

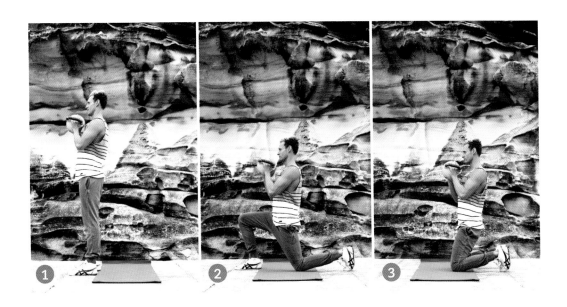

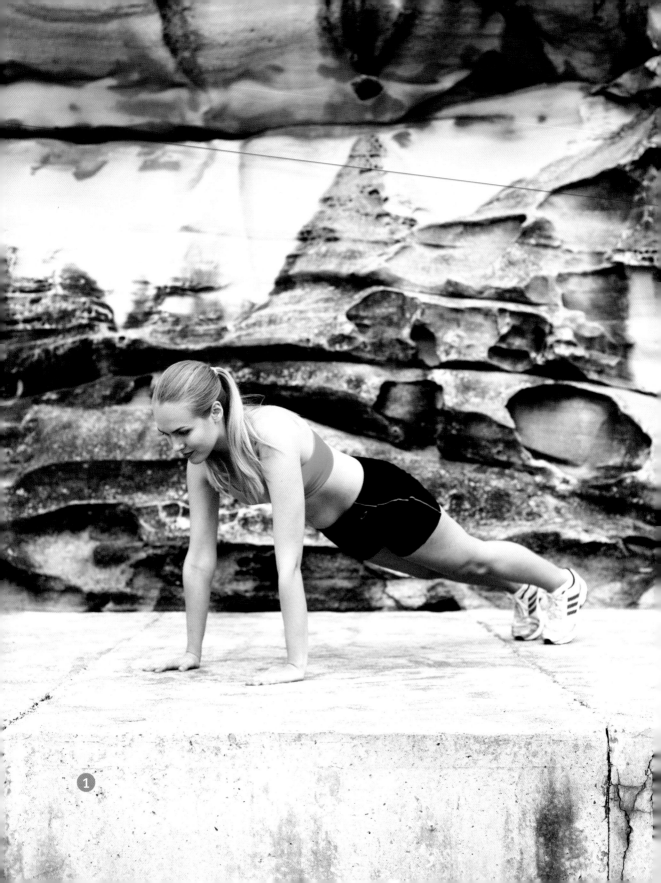

The Frog

This is a core-based exercise which requires and promotes flexibility through the hip. It's simple, but trust us – if you don't cut corners, it's full-on! A fantastic exercise, regardless of your fitness level.

Mechanics

Lie face down in a high plank. Make sure your spine is in neutral and your hands are under your shoulders.

Bring your left foot forwards, as close to the outside of your left hand as you can, and place it flat on the floor. You may find this difficult when you first try but if you persist it gets easier. The most important thing is to get a full range of movement through the hip. The tempo is slow to medium.

Hold the finish position for one to two seconds, then return the leg to the start position. Repeat with the right leg.

Variation

Harder … Insert a push-up in between each frog rep while you're in the start position.

TIP: Make sure that every frog rep takes the hip through its fullest range of motion.

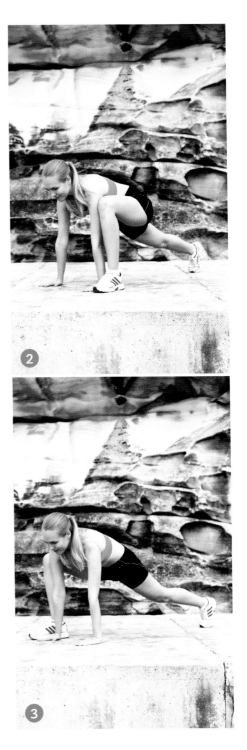

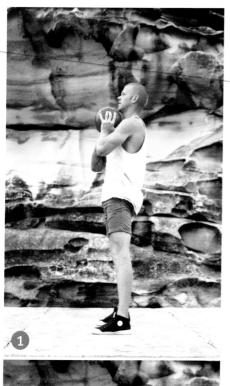

The Kettlebell Squat with Overhead Press

This is a dynamic, full-body exercise guaranteed to get you sweating and in condition in no time.

Mechanics

Stand with your feet shoulder-width apart and cup the kettlebell, holding it high against your chest, under your chin, with your elbows down.

'Break' the hip by sticking your bum out, and allow your upper body to lean forwards – but keep your back straight. Now bend your knees and lower yourself into a squat. Keep the kettlebell close to your body. All your weight should be over your heels. You should be able to wiggle your toes at the bottom of the squat.

Go as deep as you can – the lower the better – while keeping your back straight and your spine neutral. The angle of your lower leg should mirror the angle of your back. Use a mirror to check.

Rise quickly, driving your weight through your heels. Keep the kettlebell close to your chest until you are back to a standing position, then raise it above your head until your elbows are locked, or close to it. Return the kettlebell to your chest and, without pausing or stopping, descend into another squat.

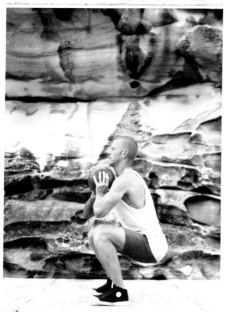

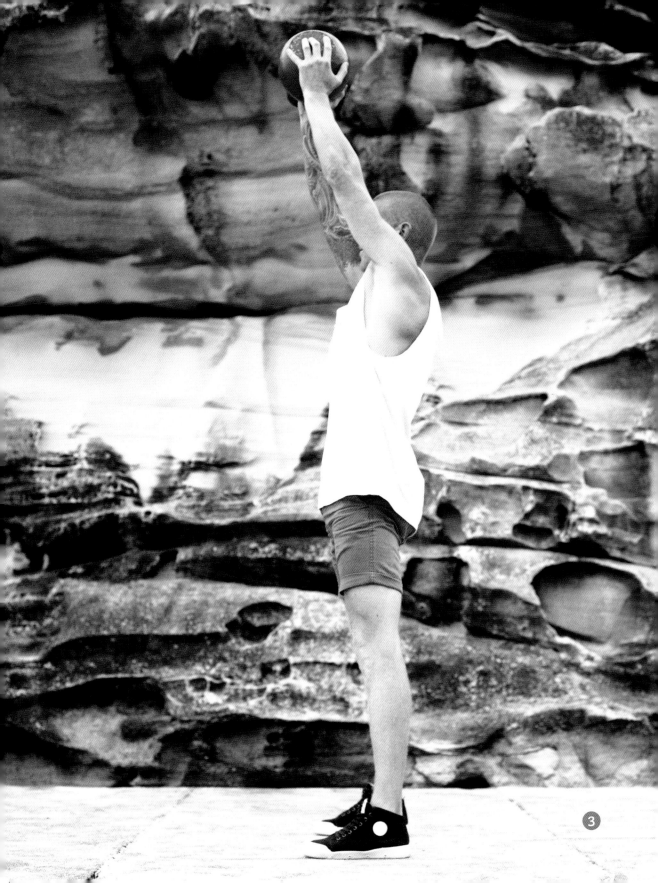

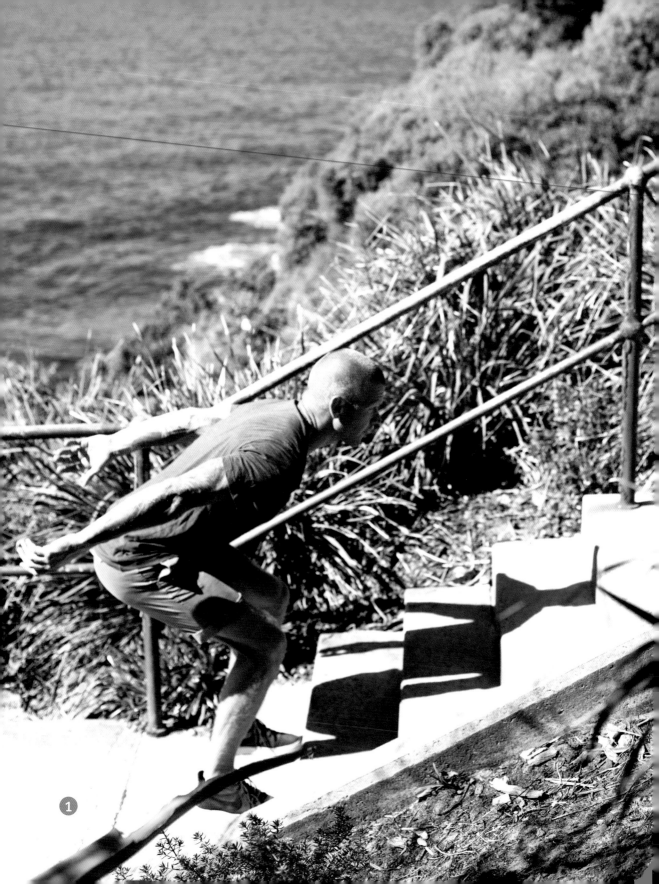

Bounding

We are big fans of bounding. There's no beating around the bush, it is hard yakka – gruelling but effective. You'll be very sore after a work-out, but you know that that means it's hitting the right spot.

Mechanics

Stand with feet shoulder-width apart, with your arms out in front at shoulder height. Sink your hips and bend your knees as you bring your arms alongside you, or even slightly behind you, and drop your weight down into your heels. Your aim is to bound forwards as far as you can, so you need to 'load up' the target muscles by stretching them initially.

Driving your arms forwards, take off with both feet. Your toes should be the last part of your foot to leave the floor. To gain maximum distance you will need maximum height.

Land on both feet and pause before bounding again, rather than performing reps in rapid succession. Each rep relies on explosive energy and demands 100 per cent exertion. Control is paramount – never compromise form.

Variation

Harder ... Incorporate stairs or steps into the exercise to increase the intensity. Choose a height that you can manage, but which challenges you without compromising form.

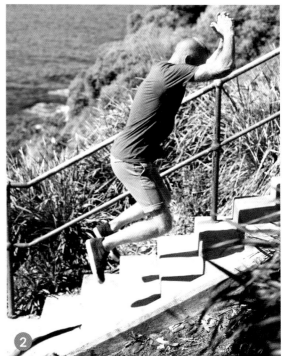

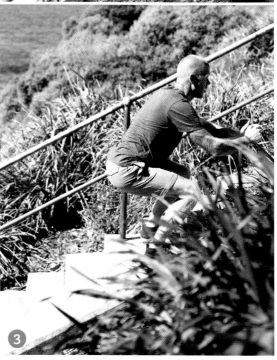

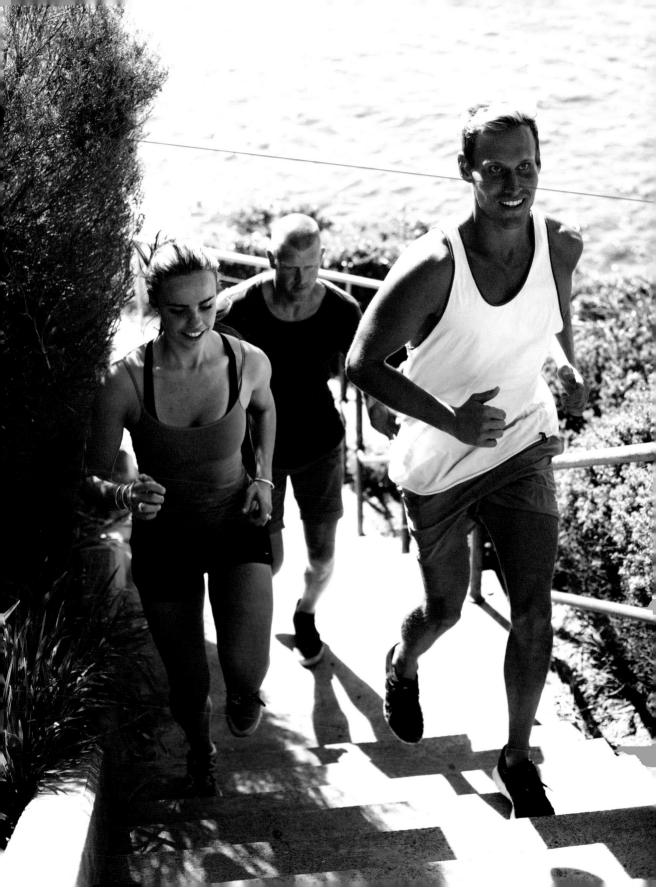

The Stairs

An often overlooked tool for strength and cardio training, stairs are accessible, free and incredibly effective in improving your cardiovascular health and toning the lower limbs. We all know that interval training is the preferred method for most trainers, and stairs provide the perfect platform. Jogging or sprinting intervals will pay dividends – although it might not feel amazing at the time.

Mechanics

Whether you're taking one, two or three steps at a time, try to stay light on your feet. Step on the balls of your feet or your forefoot. Imagine the steps are hot coals and you want to get your foot off them as quickly as possible.

Your upper body is particularly important – drive using your arms, and keep your upper body upright. Taking one step at a time will work your calves, but if you want to work your glutes as well, bend at the hip, and take two or more steps at a time. The greater the hip flexion, the more activation of the glute.

Variations

Easier … Walk like an elephant! Walking up steps like an elephant means landing on your heel, rather than the forefoot, and driving your weight down through it. The action is very deliberate and controlled. Make sure you place your entire foot on the step. Stand tall after each step before stepping forwards again.

Harder … Add weight! The upper body helps you to drive forwards and up. If you carry a medicine ball, kettlebell or dumbbell, your lower body will have to work harder to compensate.

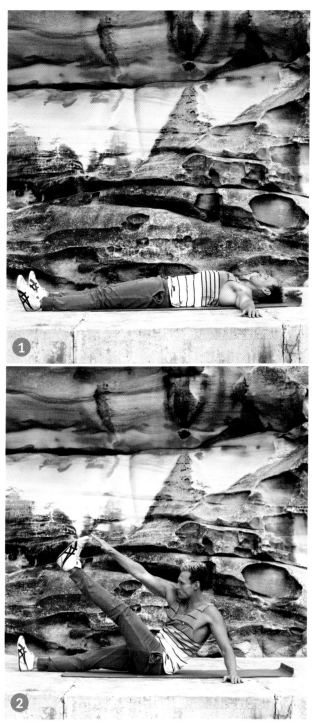

The Straight Arm & Leg Opposite Toe Tap

This is an exercise you can do lying on your back – which makes it sound easier than it really is. It's an absolute ripper of an abdominal work-out, targeting the abs and obliques. This one is guaranteed to tone your midsection.

Mechanics

Lie on your back with your feet shoulder-width apart and your arms in a crucifix position or at 45 degrees to your body above your head.

Using your left forearm as a pivot point, lift your right shoulder off the floor and bring your right hand across your body. Lift your left leg at the same time, so that you can touch your toe. You may need to bend your knee slightly, but for the best results, keep your limbs as straight as possible.

Tap your toe and return to the start position with control before performing the same action on the opposite side.

Variation

Easier ... Bending the elbow and knee joint will make the exercise easier, but as you get stronger, remember to straighten your limbs.

The Flutter Kick

This is a gem of an exercise, targeting the lower abs. You'll definitely feel the burn with this one – we know because we do!

Mechanics

Lie on your back. If it's comfortable, you can make fists with your hands and pop them under your bum. This will help keep your pelvis tilted back and your spine neutral.

Lift your heels six inches off the floor and then kick from the hips with extended knees. Keep the movement small, with an emphasis on control.

Variation

Easier ... In a tabletop position, maintain 90 degrees at the knee. Maintain tension, and try not to rest your calves on your hamstrings. Slowly extend one leg at a time and gently tap the heel on the floor, then return to the tabletop position and alternate legs.

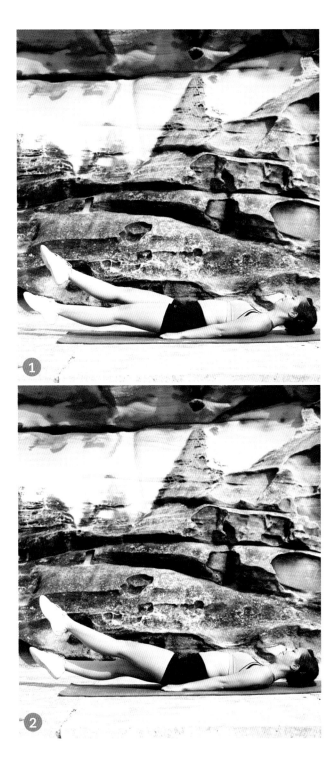

The Push-up

This is a tried-and-tested exercise for the chest and triceps. It's possibly the most recognisable exercise out there, but we certainly know how to enhance it. The humble push-up is incredibly versatile and can be used by anyone, no matter what your level of fitness.

Mechanics

Lie face down in a high plank with your hands under your shoulders and your feet together. Make sure your spine is neutral.

Squeeze your glutes and tense your abs as you bend your elbows, dipping as low as you can, then return to the start position. Maintain a solid plank position throughout the push-up, making sure your hips rise and fall at the same rate as your chest, and keeping your spine neutral.

Variations

Easier … On your knees! Rather than resting on your hands and toes, rest on your hands and knees. Keep your hips pushed forwards, create a solid plank between your knees and shoulders and ensure your hips rise and fall at the same rate as your chest.

Even easier … Work on an incline. Find a sloped surface that allows your hands to be higher than your feet.

Harder … As you dip down, let your elbows go out to the side. This changes the action of the shoulder joint and forces the target muscles in the chest to work harder.

Even harder … Give yourself a clap – make the humble push-up a real challenge and give your chest something to complain about. Drive from the lowest point of the push-up with maximum speed until your hands are off the floor. If you generate enough 'air time', clap your hands together. As you gain strength, the number of claps you can fit in will increase.

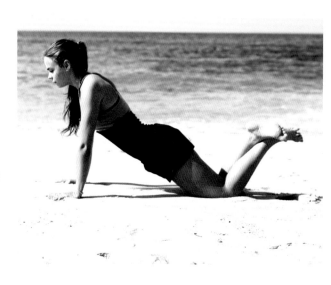

The Ultimate Push-up

The push-up is a universal exercise with numerous variations, but we think this variation has it all. It demands not only strength in your chest but also dexterity, coordination, agility and flexibility. When performed correctly, this exercise turns a humble push-up into a killer push-up, guaranteed to rip you and elicit an aerobic response. The mechanics are technical, but stick with it – it's worth it.

Mechanics

Lie face down in a high plank with your feet shoulder-width apart.

Bend your elbows and dip down as far as you can before coming back up.

As you reach the top of your push-up, take your weight on your right hand and lift your left hand off the ground. Lift your left foot off the floor at the same time.

Rotate your body, planting your left foot behind and close to your extended right knee.

Bend at the hips and try to tap your right toe with your left hand, keeping your right leg straight. This will work your abs, so resist cutting corners.

Once you have tapped your toe, return to your high plank. Do another push-up, repeating the toe tap on the opposite side.

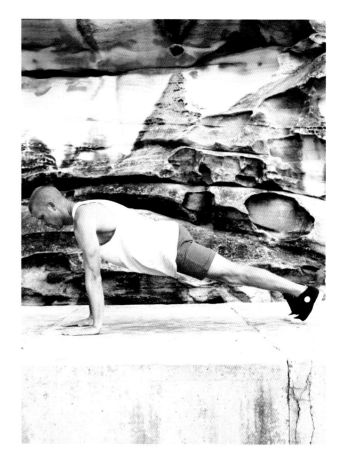

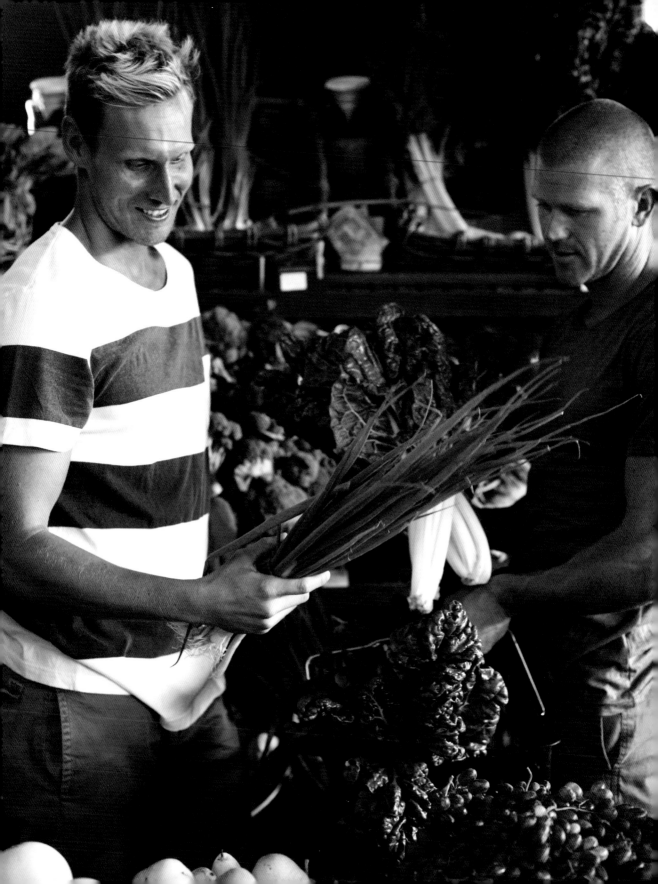

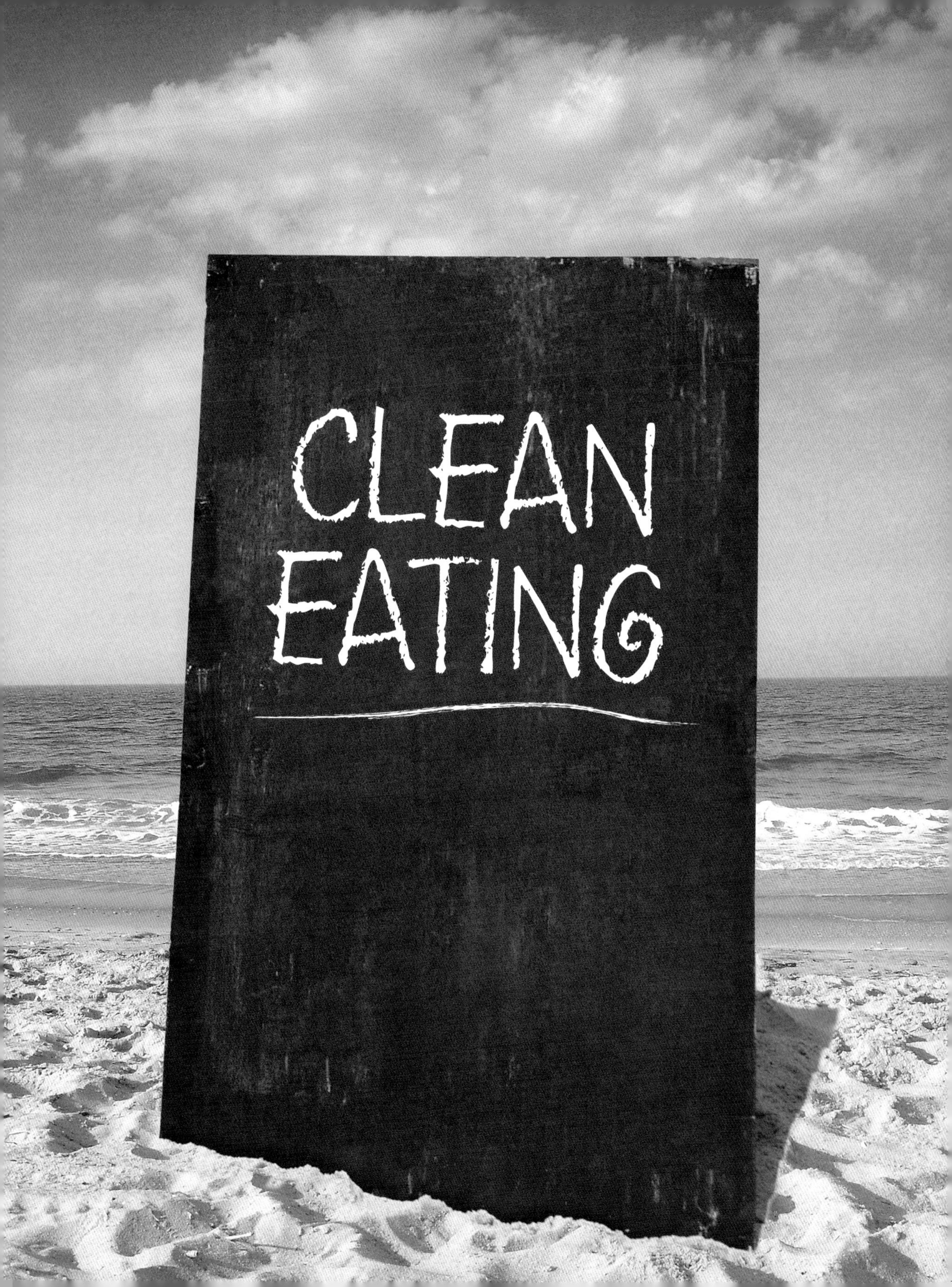
CLEAN
EATING

Making Smart Choices

We have a secret to tell you – do you want to know what it is? We are all human! Yep, that's right – we all have an off day every now and then, and sometimes we just need to eat whatever we want.

Most of us live very busy lives and there is no avoiding the fact that sometimes we cannot control what we put into our bodies. Perhaps it's a birthday dinner we're attending, and we can't find anything healthy on the menu, or maybe we're stuck between meetings and can only get some food on the run, whatever that food may be. At other times we *can* control what we eat but find ourselves craving spicy, salty or sweet snack foods. No matter what the circumstance, you can always try to make a smart choice. The following tips will help you do just that – whether you're shopping at the supermarket, eating out, or just feel like a snack at home.

Takeaway

When getting takeaway, you don't have to let your clean eating fall by the wayside. With some smart ordering you can end up with a high-protein, wholefood meal that will keep you full and satisfied. Don't be afraid to ask for what you want! Most restaurants will happily grill your food and replace chips for veggies, or put the sauce on the side of the dish so you can control how much you have. Here are a few pointers for ordering some of our favourite takeaway and restaurant meals.

Fish and Chips ... Every Friday night it was a tradition for our families to enjoy fish and chips in front of the telly. Back then we would have stuffed our faces with the greasy golden chips and deep-fried fish, but these days we order delicious grilled fish with a fresh salad.

Italian ... The Italians aren't just famous for their pizzas and pastas. Next time you're dining out at an Italian restaurant, look through the menu – you'll usually find a grilled fish, chicken or salad dish. Ask to have it with some steamed vegetables and the sauce on the side. If pizza and pasta are the only options, avoid cream-based sauces and ask if they have a gluten-free pizza base.

Japanese ... When you're eating Japanese food, don't be fooled that all of it is healthy. Try to avoid the white rice, sweet sugary sauces, deep-fried chicken and pork katsu. Instead, opt for brown rice sushi, fresh and healthy plates of sashimi, or soba noodles, made from 100 per cent buckwheat.

Mexican ... Mexican food can be healthy if you make the right choices. Steer clear of the regular corn chips and wheat-based tortillas and stick to small, soft, corn-based tacos filled with fresh ingredients like grilled chicken, avocado and salad. Ask for a little more meat to up the protein without filling up on the extras. Remember you can always ask for no cheese and no sour cream.

Thai ... With all those rich, sweet sauces, Thai food can be deceptively high in sugar. Stick to a hot and spicy tom yum soup with a green mango salad if you want to eat clean, or go for grilled cuts of meat and ask for no sauce.

Condiments, Dressings and Sauces

Some processed foods are packed full of nasties – but we don't even know it. Barbecue sauce, for example, is over 50 per cent sugar, compared to mustard, which is less than 1 per cent. Balsamic vinegar is comparatively higher in sugar than the vinegar we recommend you use – apple cider vinegar. Sweet chilli and tomato sauce are both made up of over 45 per cent sugar. We love dressings made up of avocado oil, mustard, apple cider vinegar and lemon juice. Or try tamari when cooking Asian – it tastes great and contains very little sugar. When cooking, swap olive oil for coconut oil. Coconut oil is a fantastic energy source and is stable when heated, meaning it doesn't turn into a nasty fat.

Dairy

We highly recommend you avoid eating low-fat products. Low-fat dairy products don't taste as good as the full-fat versions, so the fat is often replaced with sugar to make them taste better. If you eat milk and yogurt, always choose the full-fat varieties for optimal health.

Smart Snack Swaps

When you are craving something sweet or fatty, try one of our smart snack swaps:

Chocolate bar > our Cacao-nut Crunch Clusters (see page 116)
Potato chips > our Sweet Potato Fries (see page 125)
Milkshake > our Green, Lean and Clean Smoothie (see page 78)
Soft drink > Fresh lime in mineral water

We're always told that breakfast is the most important meal of the day. Well, it is true – the word 'breakfast' itself broken down means 'break the fast'. You have been without food overnight as you sleep and it's important to give your body the metabolic kick it needs to get your day off to an energetic, focused start. But that doesn't mean filling up your body with empty calories and sugar-laden cereals.

Many of us have been taught that a 'healthy breakfast' consists of starch-based foods, predominantly cereals, muffins and bread, and foods containing high amounts of sugar, such as fruit juice. We want to dispel the myth that you need to fuel up on heavy, wheat-based carbohydrates first thing in the morning. Instead, turbocharge your day with high-protein foods that are high in good fats to keep your body healthy inside and out.

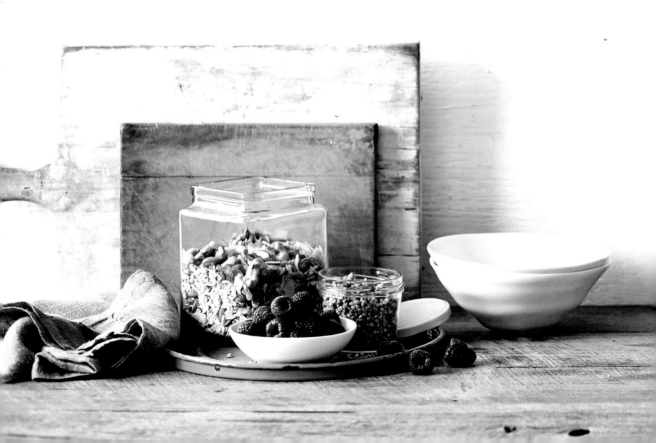

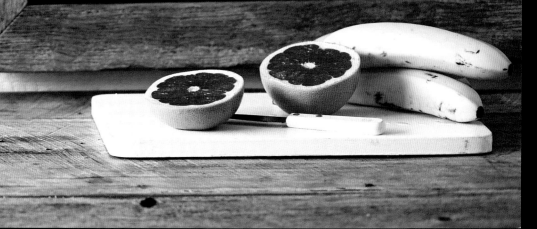

BREAKFAST

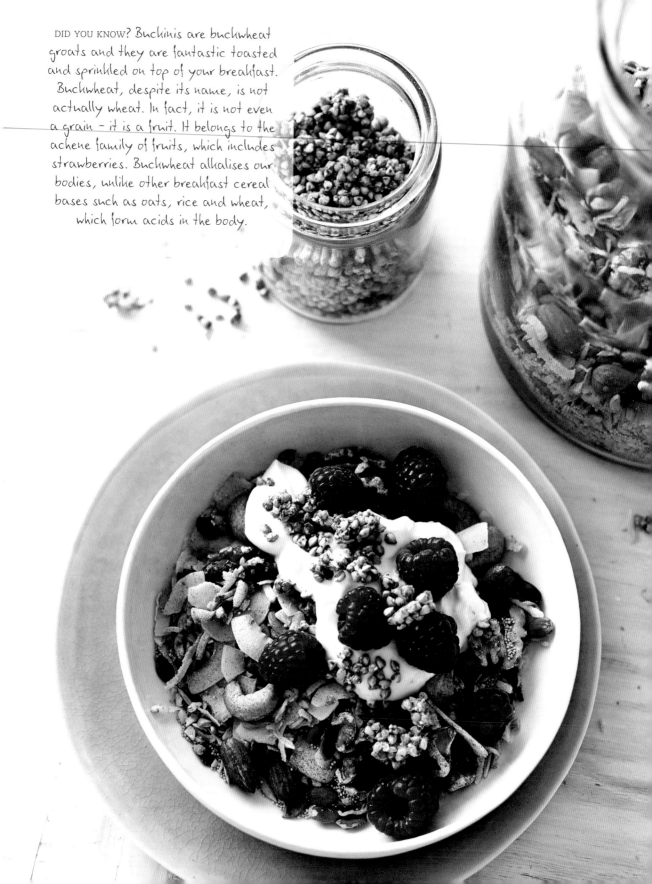

DID YOU KNOW? Buchinis are buckwheat groats and they are fantastic toasted and sprinkled on top of your breakfast. Buckwheat, despite its name, is not actually wheat. In fact, it is not even a grain – it is a fruit. It belongs to the achene family of fruits, which includes strawberries. Buckwheat alkalises our bodies, unlike other breakfast cereal bases such as oats, rice and wheat, which form acids in the body.

Surf-side Granola with Raspberries

Serves 4

We love this recipe because it brings breakfast back to basics. It's homemade, all natural, and the coconut flakes remind us of the beach. The smell of it while baking gives you that healthy feeling inside and makes the house smell great! We love to eat this with unsweetened dairy-free coconut yoghurt.

2 cups coconut flakes

1 cup amaranth seeds

½ cup activated almonds (see recipe on page 115)

½ cup raw cashews

½ cup walnuts

½ cup sunflower seeds

½ cup raw pepitas (dried pumpkin seeds)

2 tablespoons chia seeds

1 teaspoon cinnamon

2 teaspoons coconut oil, melted

1 teaspoon rice malt syrup

coconut yoghurt, to serve

fresh raspberries, to serve

toasted buckinis, to garnish

1. Preheat oven to 180°C and prepare 2 baking trays with baking paper.

2. In a bowl, mix the dry ingredients and stir in the coconut oil and rice malt syrup. Evenly distribute the mix across the trays and bake for 15 minutes, or until golden and crunchy, swapping trays halfway during cooking and tossing ingredients.

3. Set aside and allow to cool, then serve with coconut yoghurt and fresh raspberries, with toasted buckinis as a garnish on top.

NOTE: This is a great recipe to make in large batches. Preparation is key to any healthy lifestyle, so be prepared and whip up a big batch ahead of time. You can mix and match your ingredient quantities to get your favourite flavours spot-on. Package some up in an old jam jar and give it as a gift to your friends.

Amaranth and Chia Porridge

Serves 4

This dish is a delicious winter warmer, rich in flavour and high in fibre. Chia seeds are great because they contain high levels of omega-3 fatty acids. They can reduce sugar cravings and help you feel fuller, longer.

2 cups amaranth seeds, soaked overnight

4 tablespoons chia seeds

500 ml coconut milk

pinch of sea salt

pinch of nutmeg

pinch of ground ginger

pinch of cinnamon

1 vanilla bean, scraped, or 1 teaspoon vanilla extract

rice malt syrup (optional)

freshly toasted shredded coconut, to garnish

2 fresh figs, quartered

1. Drain and rinse the amaranth seeds. In a saucepan, combine the amaranth, chia seeds, coconut milk, salt, spices and vanilla. Bring to the boil, then turn the heat to low and allow to simmer gently for 20–25 minutes, stirring regularly. Add some water if it's looking a little dry.

2. Remove from heat and set aside, covered, for 10 minutes or so. (The longer it stands the thicker it becomes, but you can always add a little more water or coconut milk if needed.)

3. Drizzle with a little rice malt syrup, if desired, and garnish with shredded coconut. Serve with the fresh figs.

VARIATION: Oats are classed as a grain, so they're not usually considered 'paleo', but we believe they offer important health benefits. They are low GI, high in fibre and help lower cholesterol. They are also affordable and widely available. Oats make a good substitute for amaranth in this recipe if you are having trouble finding amaranth.

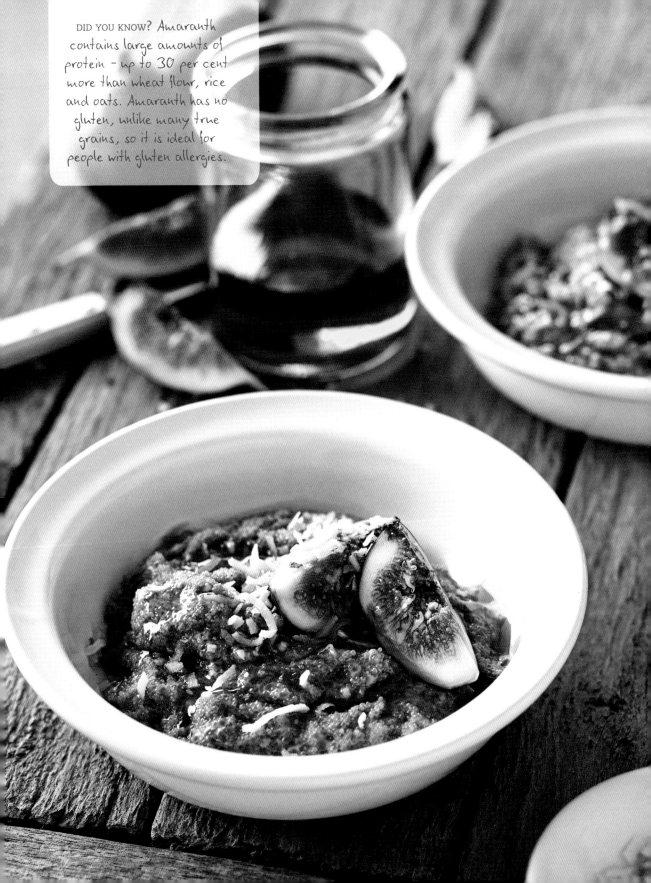

DID YOU KNOW? Amaranth contains large amounts of protein – up to 30 per cent more than wheat flour, rice and oats. Amaranth has no gluten, unlike many true grains, so it is ideal for people with gluten allergies.

DID YOU KNOW? Chia seeds are a fantastic source of essential fatty acids and are a great addition to a healthy diet. The seeds come in black or white and both are highly nutritious. They can help reduce blood pressure, stabilise blood sugar and give you a massive boost of energy, which is why Aztec warriors used them before heading into battle.

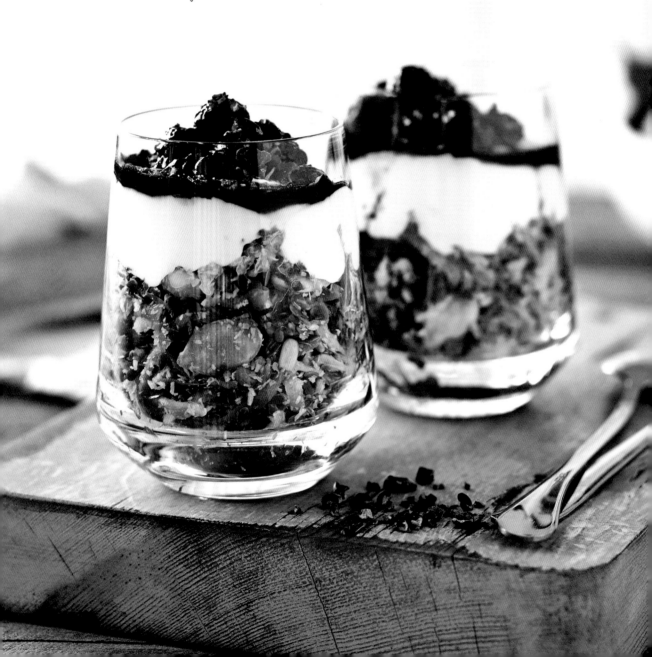

Paleo Parfait

Serves 4

One of the struggles with paleo-style breakfasts is finding a suitable substitute for your old favourites like Bircher muesli and regular packet cereals, which are usually sugar-laden and high in gluten and wheat. This parfait is a great breakfast treat that tastes as good as it looks.

½ cup sesame seeds

½ cup pepitas

½ cup sunflower seeds

½ cup golden flaxseeds

½ cup activated almonds (see recipe on page 115)

½ cup desiccated coconut

1 cup frozen mixed berries

1 tablespoon rice malt syrup

1 apple, grated

1 large carrot, grated

coconut cream, to serve

cocoa nibs, to garnish

VARIATION: If you want to try something different, head out to your local health-food store and pick up some coconut yoghurt. It is gluten, dairy and sugar free, tastes great and is an awesome substitute for coconut cream.

1. Preheat oven to 180°C and prepare 2 baking trays with baking paper. On one tray, toast the seeds for about 15 minutes, until golden and crunchy. On the second tray, toast the almonds and coconut for 8–10 minutes. Watch both trays, as they take different amounts of time to cook, and you do not want to burn them. Once the ingredients are toasted, combine well and set aside to cool slightly.

2. Meanwhile, in a medium saucepan, combine the frozen berries and rice malt syrup and soften over low to medium heat, until they reach a sauce-like consistency. Mash a few of the berries up if you'd like to create more of a puree, then set aside.

3. Combine the grated apple and carrot with the toasted seed mixture and you're ready to plate up.

4. In a glass, gradually layer to your liking, perhaps starting with berries, then seeds, then berries again. Top with a dollop of coconut cream and garnish with some cocoa nibs.

Banana and Quinoa Porridge

Serves 4

This is a hearty, gluten-free porridge that is quick to make and warms you perfectly on those cool, fresh mornings. It will keep you full all the way to lunch, so you won't be tempted to reach for any of those naughty midmorning treats.

500 ml almond milk

1 cup quinoa flakes

1 ripe banana, sliced

1 vanilla bean, scraped

1 tablespoon chia seeds

pinch of cinnamon

toasted activated almonds,
  crushed, to garnish (see
  recipe on page 115)

1 tablespoon rice malt syrup

1. Combine the almond milk and 500 ml water in a saucepan and bring to a simmer over medium heat.
2. Add the quinoa flakes, banana and vanilla. Cook until thickened, stirring often.
3. Add the chia seeds and stir through.
4. Sprinkle with some cinnamon and crushed almonds, and drizzle with the rice malt syrup.

NOTE: Rice malt syrup is a great alternative to regular sweeteners. It is a natural sweetener, made from fermented cooked rice. You can usually find it in health-food stores and some supermarkets. One teaspoon of sugar is equivalent to one teaspoon of rice malt syrup.

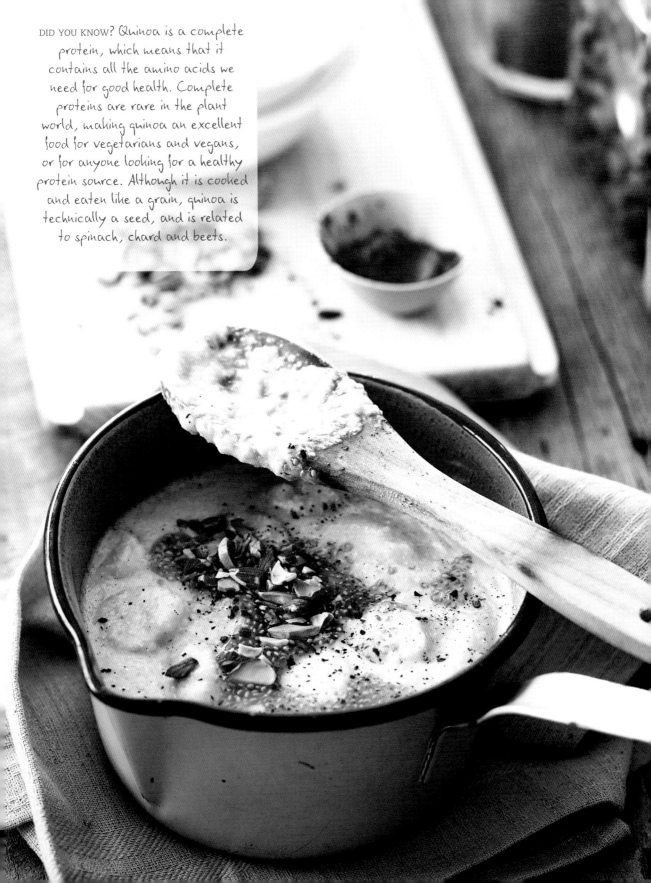

DID YOU KNOW? Quinoa is a complete protein, which means that it contains all the amino acids we need for good health. Complete proteins are rare in the plant world, making quinoa an excellent food for vegetarians and vegans, or for anyone looking for a healthy protein source. Although it is cooked and eaten like a grain, quinoa is technically a seed, and is related to spinach, chard and beets.

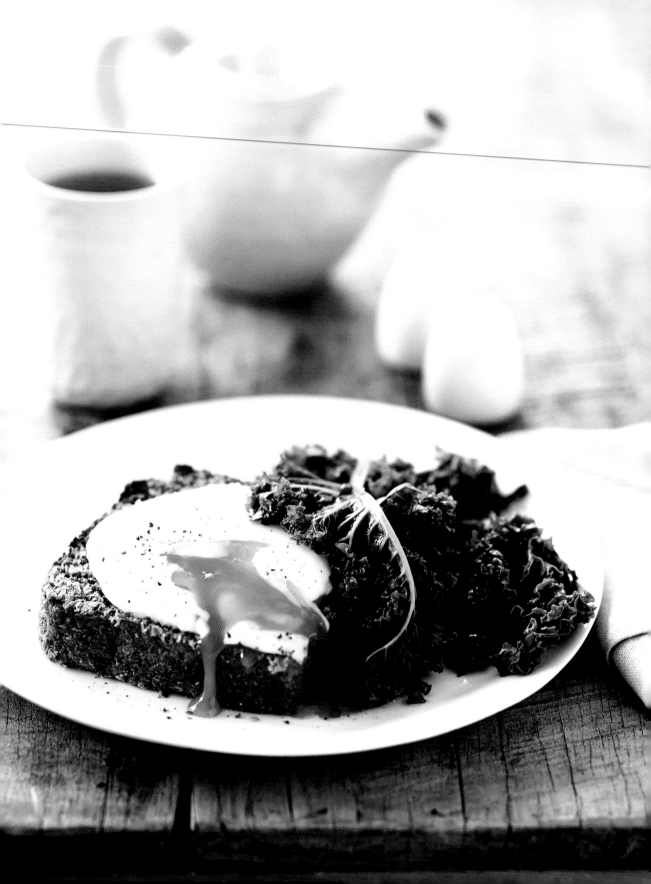

Perfect Poached Eggs

Serves as many as you like!

There's nothing better than that feeling of cutting into a freshly poached egg to see the yolk ooze out all over your plate. It's what we go to cafes for on the weekend. Now it's time to do it at home so you can have a protein-rich breakfast, any day of the week. Eggs are also a wonderful addition to any meal because they are so versatile and go with pretty much anything. If we eat out at a cafe and the salad doesn't have enough protein, sometimes we order an egg to go on top.

eggs

1–2 teaspoons white vinegar

THE ADD-ONS: Eggs make a delicious breakfast, but what can we have with them? Here are just a few ideas.

SPROUTED TOAST: With so many people not eating wheat or processed breads, we recommend tracking down a good-quality sprouted loaf.

KALE: This superfood is packed full of iron, calcium and antioxidants, and makes a great base for perfectly poached eggs. Just sauté in a frying pan with a teaspoon of coconut oil and allow it to soften. Add some freshly chopped chilli and some pink salt and you're ready to go.

1. Fill a small saucepan with about 10 cm of water and bring to the boil. Add just a teaspoon or so of vinegar to help the eggs stay in one piece and not go all over the place.

2. Crack an egg and place it carefully on a large, slotted spoon which allows the watery membrane to drip off the main part of the egg white. Create a small whirlpool in the water with a spoon, then lower the egg on the slotted spoon into the centre of the just boiling water. The egg should stay together as it cooks.

3. Poach for a few minutes, until the yolk has reached the desired consistency. We like to watch closely and remove it with the slotted spoon when it's still soft in the centre.

Shakshuka with Crispy Bacon

Serves 4

Shakshuka is an awesome-tasting Middle Eastern–style breakfast. The eggs are poached in the thick spicy sauce, and the bacon on top adds a delicious saltiness to the dish.

coconut oil, for frying

1 small red onion, finely chopped

1 garlic clove, minced

1 red capsicum, seeded and chopped

2 teaspoons tomato paste

1 teaspoon ground cumin

1 teaspoon chilli powder

1 teaspoon sweet paprika

pinch of cayenne pepper

6 medium-sized tomatoes, diced

sea salt and ground black pepper

8 eggs (2 per person)

4 rashers middle bacon

avocado, to garnish

flat-leaf parsley, to garnish

1. Place a large frying pan over medium heat, add the coconut oil and allow it to melt. Add the red onion and sauté for about two minutes, or until softened. Mix in the garlic and continue to cook until the onion becomes tender and slightly golden. Be careful not to burn the garlic or it will give the dish a bitter taste. Add the red capsicum to the pan and mix well. Sauté for about 5 minutes, just until the capsicum is tender.

2. Add the tomato paste to the pan, followed by the cumin, chilli powder, paprika and cayenne pepper. Fry this off for a minute and then add the tomatoes. Give the mixture a taste and add more spices, if you like, along with salt and pepper. Simmer over low heat, covered, for 15 minutes. The longer it simmers, the richer the sauce becomes.

3. Create small 'indents' in the tomato mixture with a spoon, making sure they are spaced evenly, then crack the eggs into them. Cover the pan and cook for between 10 and 15 minutes, or until the eggs turn white and no clear liquids run.

4. Once the eggs have cooked through, fry up some bacon in a separate pan and place it on top of the eggs to give the dish height and colour. Thinly slice some avocado over the top to get those good fats in your diet, then garnish with fresh parsley.

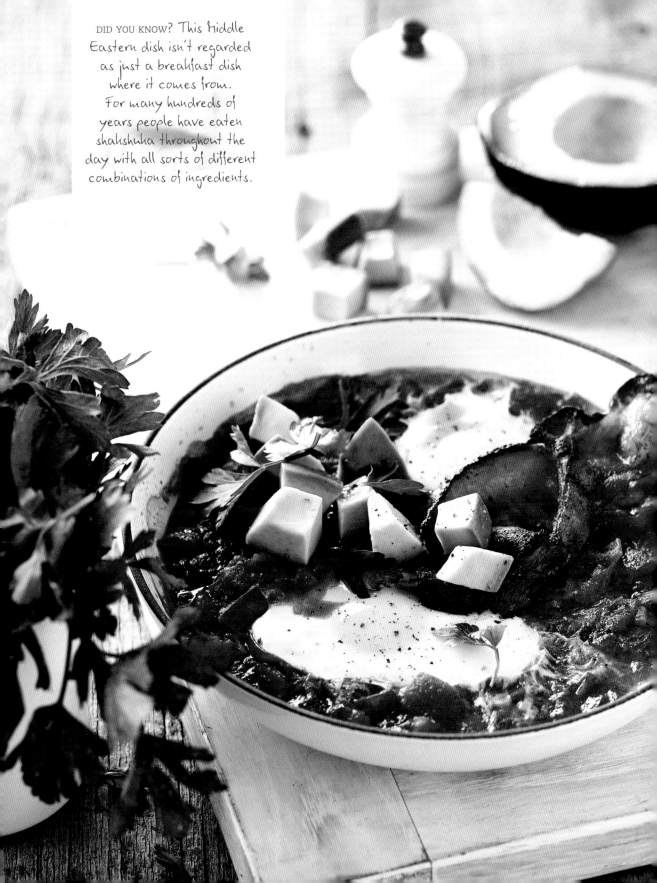

DID YOU KNOW? This Middle Eastern dish isn't regarded as just a breakfast dish where it comes from. For many hundreds of years people have eaten shakshuka throughout the day with all sorts of different combinations of ingredients.

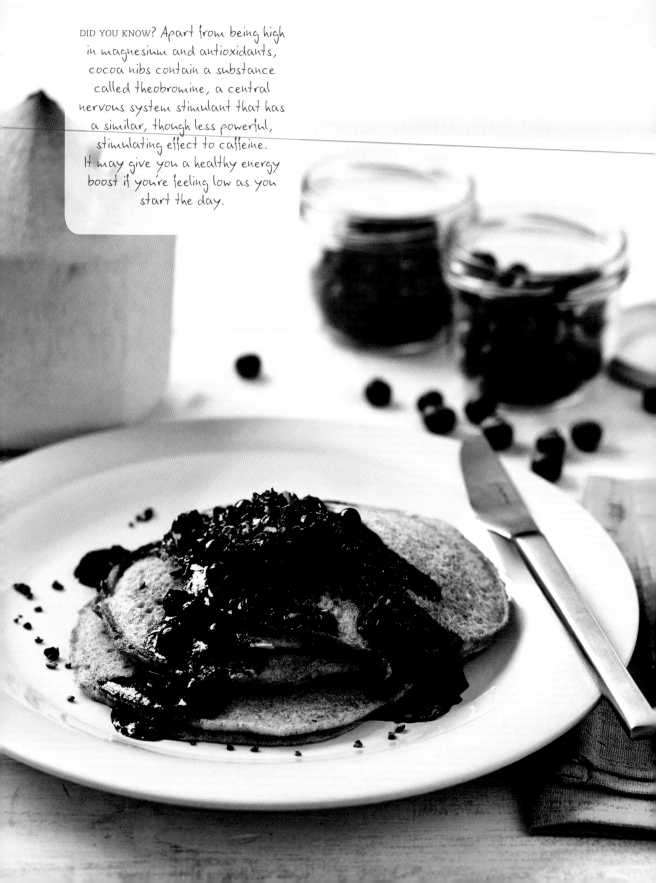

DID YOU KNOW? Apart from being high in magnesium and antioxidants, cocoa nibs contain a substance called theobromine, a central nervous system stimulant that has a similar, though less powerful, stimulating effect to caffeine. It may give you a healthy energy boost if you're feeling low as you start the day.

Coconut Pancakes with Blueberry Coulis

Serves 4

Yes, you can eat pancakes and still be healthy! They just have to be free of sugar and high in protein. These pancakes are a great example of a paleo recipe, as they really highlight the versatility of coconuts. This recipe is a great one for the weekend, when you want to relax and unwind and feel like having a bit of a treat.

4 eggs, whisked

2 × 400 ml cans coconut milk

⅓ cup coconut oil, just melted, plus extra for frying

½ cup coconut flour

1½ cups buckwheat flour

2 teaspoons baking powder

1 vanilla bean, scraped

zest of 1 orange, finely grated

pinch of sea salt

½ cup desiccated coconut

cocoa nibs, to garnish

Blueberry coulis

1 cup blueberries (fresh or frozen)

1 teaspoon rice malt syrup (optional)

1 tablespoon butter

1 teaspoon cinnamon

1 teaspoon vanilla extract

1. Combine the eggs, coconut milk and coconut oil and mix well. Gradually add the dry ingredients, making sure everything is well combined. If the mixture is looking too thick, add a little water to loosen.

2. Heat a little coconut oil in a large frying pan over medium heat. Cook the pancakes until golden on each side, turning once. This mixture makes about 12 pancakes. The key with pancakes is waiting for bubbles to appear on the top before flipping them over.

3. To make the coulis, mix the blueberries, rice malt syrup (if using), butter, cinnamon and vanilla together in a saucepan and bring to the boil, slightly mashing the blueberries, and cooking until it reaches a consistency you like. Allow to cool slightly before pouring over your pancakes. Top your breakfast with cocoa nibs for crunch, texture and that superfood hit!

VARIATION: Toasted nuts and seeds add great texture to this dish. Toast some activated almonds (see recipe on page 115) or pepitas and sprinkle on top to create a beautiful, nutrient-dense topping.

Green, Lean and Clean Smoothie

Serves 2

This smoothie is great when you need a nutrient kick. It's packed full of healthy ingredients that will keep you nourished while making you feel full at the same time. You can mix up the ingredients depending on what you have in your fridge. The egg and cashews add a protein hit to make this a complete meal.

½ lemon, peeled and with pith and seeds removed

½ green apple, cored

1 cucumber, roughly chopped

½ cup frozen sliced banana

½ cup kale, stems removed

½ cup mint

1 raw egg

2 tablespoons raw cashews

250 ml coconut water

It's as simple as combining all the ingredients in a good blender and mixing until you've achieved your desired consistency. This will make a couple of cups' worth, so share the green love.

TIP: We like to make this smoothie with the addition of a high-quality whey or pea protein, and a greens powder. Ask your local health-food store for good products that you can add to this mix to really amp it up.

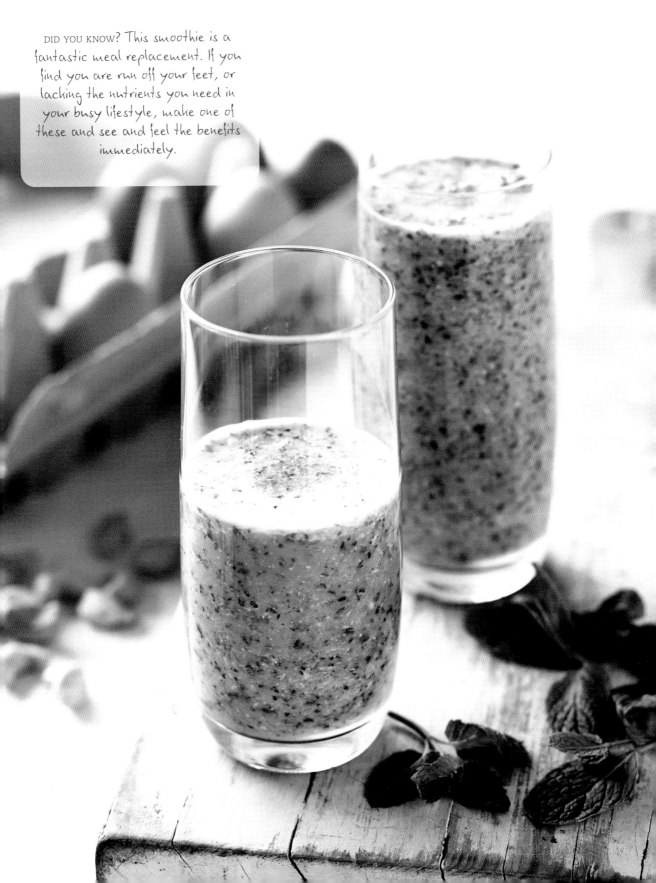

DID YOU KNOW? This smoothie is a fantastic meal replacement. If you find you are run off your feet, or lacking the nutrients you need in your busy lifestyle, make one of these and see and feel the benefits immediately.

After you have started your day with a nutrient-dense breakfast, lunch is your next major opportunity to fuel your body and mind for the remainder of the day. What you eat will be reflected in your mood and energy levels, which means it is smart to choose fresh, clean food that gives you sustained energy and keeps you feeling full.

When deciding what to have for lunch, preparation is certainly key. It pays to plan ahead and think about what leftovers from dinner can be turned into lunch the next day. It's also great to sit down and plan your lunches at the start of the week. Make a shopping list, get all the greens and whip up some meals in bulk that can be divided into separate containers to store in the fridge or freezer.

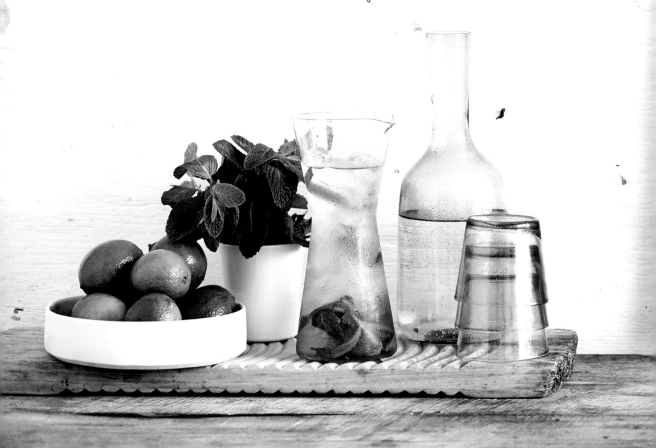

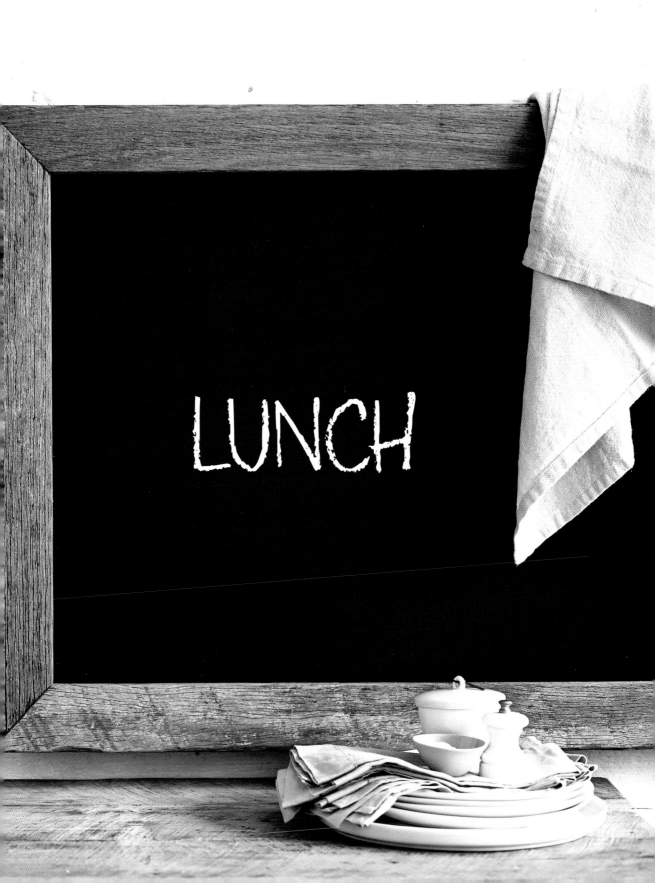

DID YOU KNOW? We absolutely love coconut oil. It offers fantastic health benefits and is the only oil we cook with these days. Lots of people are initially scared off because it is a saturated fat, but not all saturated fats are created equal. Coconut oil contains short-term, medium-chain saturated fatty acids, which are metabolised by our liver, immediately converting them into energy rather than being stored for fat. In addition, coconut oil has been proven to control weight, manage type-2 diabetes, and support immunity. You can take a teaspoon with your morning smoothie or use it as cooking oil.

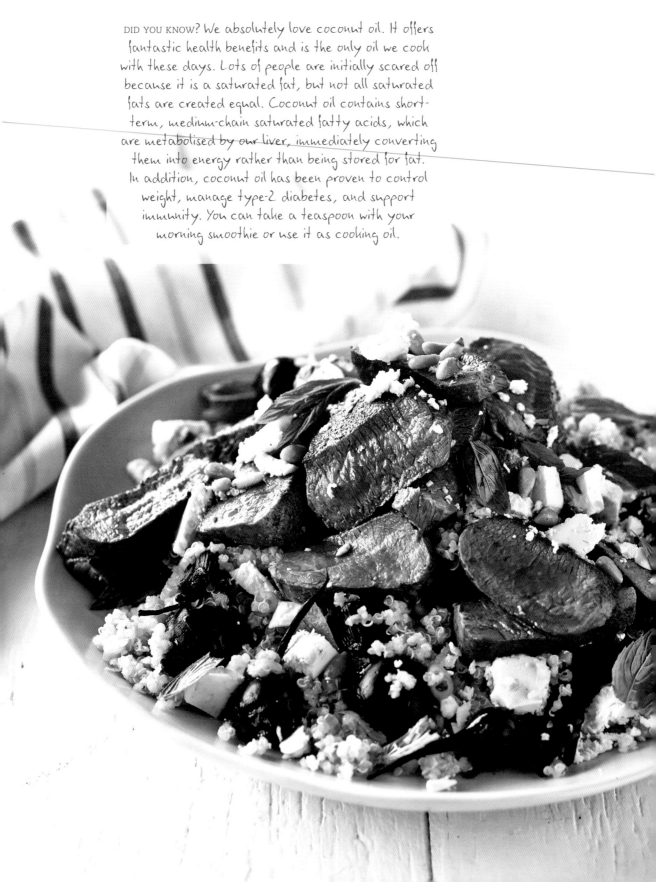

Chilli Lamb and Quinoa Salad with Roast Beetroot, Feta and Toasted Pine Nuts

Serves 4

This is an awesome salad that can be prepared in a large batch and used for a number of meals. Everything keeps really well in the fridge, and it is good eaten hot or cold.

4 baby beetroots (about 160 g in total)

2 teaspoons chilli flakes, crushed

1 teaspoon sea salt

1 tablespoon coconut oil

4 lamb loins (800 g in total)

1 cup cooked quinoa (see recipe on page 118)

30 g goat's feta

2 tablespoons pine nuts, toasted

1 tablespoon avocado oil, plus extra to drizzle

1 tablespoon finely chopped spring onion

⅓ cup torn mint leaves

juice and zest of 1 lemon, zest finely grated

1. Preheat oven to 180°C. Wrap the beetroots in foil and roast for 40 minutes, or until soft and tender. Leave them to cool, then peel and chop into halves or quarters. Set aside.
2. Pound the chilli flakes using a mortar and pestle until you have a fine powder. Add the sea salt and rub the meat well with this mixture.
3. Bring a large frying pan up to high heat with the coconut oil, then add the meat and sear well until the outside is caramelised and a nice golden-brown colour. Allow the lamb to rest for 5 minutes before slicing.
4. Combine the beets, quinoa, feta, pine nuts and avocado oil, then top with sliced lamb, spring onion, mint and lemon juice and zest. Drizzle with extra avocado oil just before serving.

VARIATION: This salad can easily be transformed into a vegetarian option. Try substituting the lamb with some extra vegetables like chargrilled zucchini and capsicum.

Spicy Kangaroo Burgers Stacked with Sweet Potato Fritters and Sautéed Kale

Serves 4

We love this! It is truly the quintessential healthy burger. We have replaced the bread with sweet potato fritters and whacked in some super-healthy sautéed kale.

1 tablespoon coriander seeds

1 tablespoon cumin seeds

600 g kangaroo mince

2 garlic cloves, crushed

1 eschalot, finely chopped or grated

2 eggs

1 small red chilli, deseeded and finely chopped

sea salt and ground black pepper

2 large sweet potatoes (about 1 kg in total)

1 cup fresh coriander, finely chopped

coconut oil, for frying

1 bunch fresh kale, stems removed and leaves torn in half

VARIATION: You can really mix and match with these burgers. Fresh lettuce, tomato and relish are great additions.

1. Heat the cumin and coriander seeds in a small pan over medium heat until they pop and become fragrant. Remove them from the heat, let them cool, then crush them up with a mortar and pestle.

2. In a large bowl place the mince, garlic and eschalot, using your hands to combine the ingredients. Add the crushed seeds, one of the eggs, the chilli, salt and pepper.

3. Shape the mince mixture into 4 equal-sized patties and (if you have the time) chill the patties for 15 minutes to help them firm up before cooking.

4. Heat a barbecue or non-stick frying pan and add some coconut oil. Cook the patties until golden on the outside and just cooked in the middle.

5. While the patties are cooking, prepare the fritters. Grate the sweet potatoes into a bowl and add the coriander and some salt and pepper. Stir through the remaining egg to bind it all together, then dollop out spoonfuls of the mixture into a hot frying pan coated with coconut oil (makes 8 to 12 fritters). Flatten them down slightly and cook until golden and crispy. Set them aside.

6. Just before serving your stack, sauté some kale in a little bit of coconut oil until softened, then layer the kangaroo burgers with the fritters and the kale.

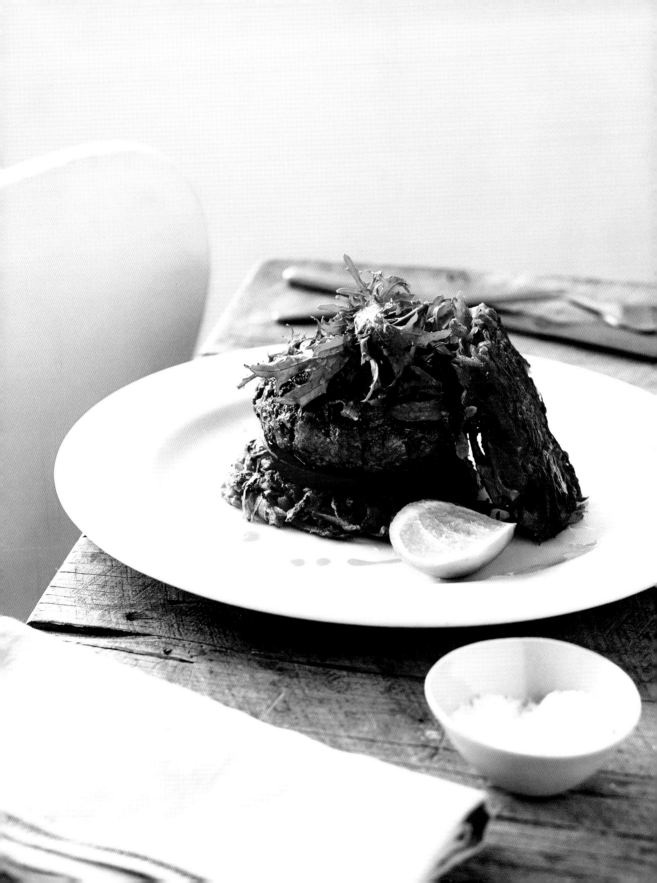

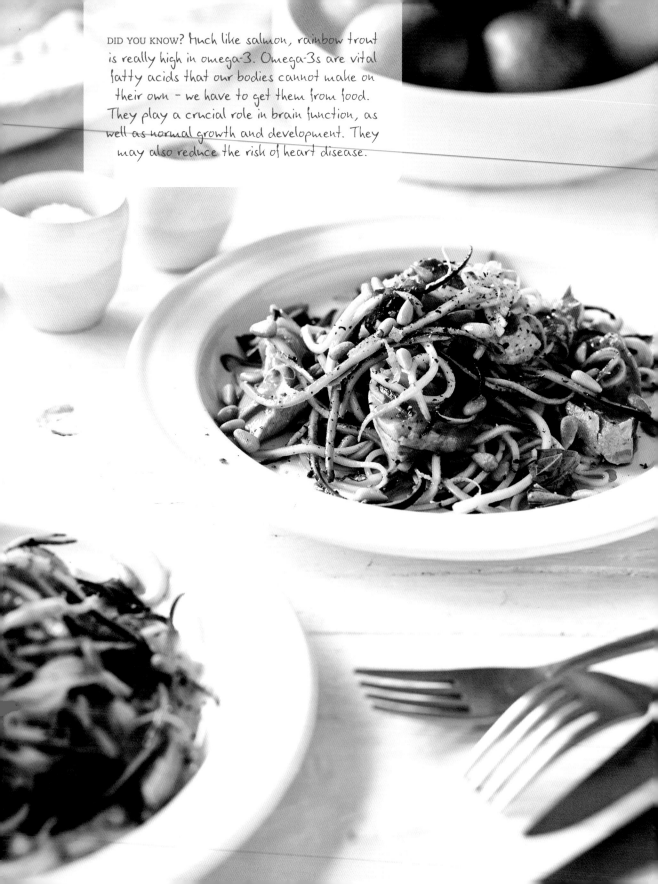

DID YOU KNOW? Much like salmon, rainbow trout is really high in omega-3. Omega-3s are vital fatty acids that our bodies cannot make on their own – we have to get them from food. They play a crucial role in brain function, as well as normal growth and development. They may also reduce the risk of heart disease.

Zucchini Linguine with Poached Rainbow Trout

Serves 4

We love making a pasta dish out of vegetables! We turn the humble zucchini into the pasta in this dish – it's so easy to do, and great for your health. Rainbow trout is rich in colour and texture, and, when poached, just perfect to toss through the linguine.

4 large zucchini

⅓ cup avocado oil, plus 1 tablespoon extra

½ cup torn fresh basil leaves

juice and zest of 1 lemon, zest finely grated

a pinch of sea salt

400 g rainbow trout fillets, boned and skin removed

½ cup pine nuts, toasted

1. Julienne the zucchini in a food processor, or use a potato peeler to shave off long, thin slices, then cut into thin strips to create the pasta.
2. Blanch the zucchini in salted boiling water just until the water comes back up to the boil, then drain, rinse and toss in a bowl with the avocado oil, basil leaves, lemon juice and salt.
3. Place the rainbow trout fillets in a pot of already boiled water, put the lid on and sit it on the bench. Remove the fish after 5–8 minutes, depending on how well done you like your fish.
4. Drain the fish and flake it apart gently with a fork. Toss with the zucchini pasta, lemon zest, extra avocado oil and toasted pine nuts.

VARIATION: You can try all sorts of different fish with this dish. We make it with salmon as well. For a vegetarian option, omit the fish and add a beautiful kale pesto.

Luke and Scott's Niçoise

Serves 4

The combination of tuna, eggs and white anchovies makes this salad a protein hit. We love how fresh this dish is, and how easy it is to take to work or enjoy as a large platter with friends on the weekend. It's vibrant and colourful, and makes you feel great.

1 punnet (250 g) cherry tomatoes, halved

2 tablespoons avocado oil

coconut oil, for frying

4 small pieces of sashimi-grade tuna (500 g in total)

sea salt and ground black pepper

180 g asparagus, trimmed and cut into 5 cm lengths

50 g rocket leaves

juice of 1 lemon

1 tablespoon raw apple cider vinegar

2 eggs, soft boiled, shelled and quartered

100 g white anchovies

1. Preheat oven to 200°C. Drizzle the cherry tomatoes with 1 tablespoon of the avocado oil and roast them for about 10–12 minutes, or until they are soft and tender and just starting to brown up.

2. Season the tuna with salt and pepper. Heat a large frying pan with coconut oil, and when the pan is nice and hot, just sear the tuna pieces quickly on each side until they're a good colour but not cooked through. You want the tuna to be rare on the inside with a thin layer of brown on the outside. Remove the tuna from the pan and set aside to rest.

3. Get the asparagus ready by blanching it in boiling water for a minute or so, then running it under cold water to stop the cooking process.

4. To make the salad, flake the tuna in a bowl and add the roasted tomatoes, asparagus and rocket. Whisk together the remaining avocado oil with the lemon juice and vinegar for the dressing.

5. Place the salad on large plates or in bowls, then top with the egg, white anchovies, dressing and salt and pepper to taste.

VARIATION: You can always use a good-quality tinned tuna or salmon for this salad. We love sustainably caught tuna and salmon in spring water.

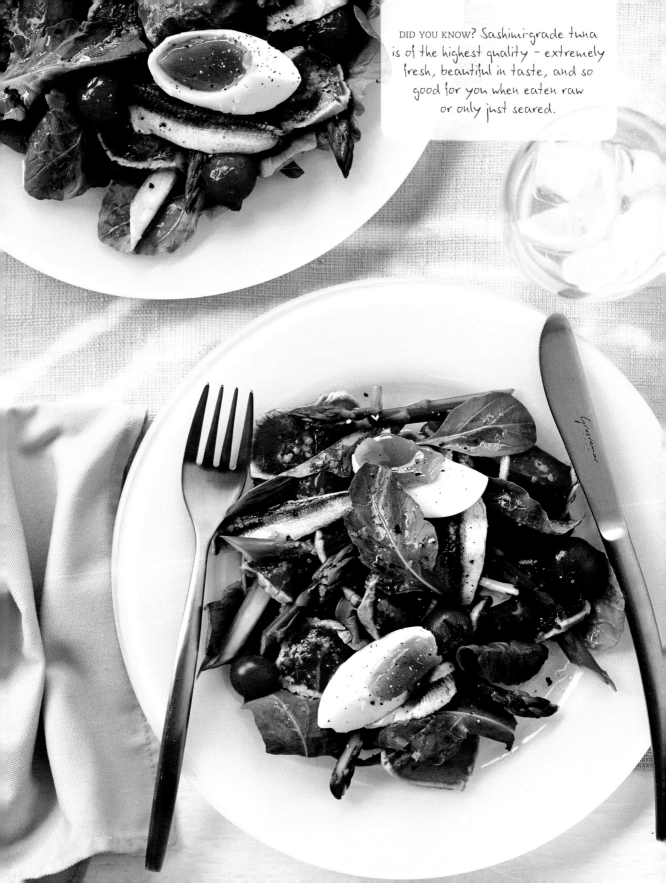

DID YOU KNOW? Sashimi-grade tuna is of the highest quality – extremely fresh, beautiful in taste, and so good for you when eaten raw or only just seared.

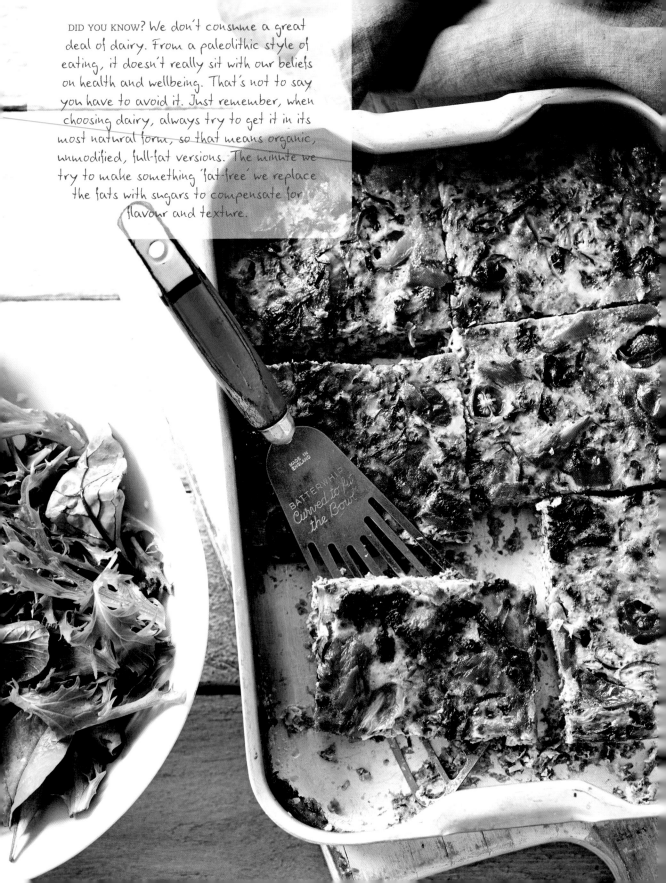

DID YOU KNOW? We don't consume a great deal of dairy. From a paleolithic style of eating, it doesn't really sit with our beliefs on health and wellbeing. That's not to say you have to avoid it. Just remember, when choosing dairy, always try to get it in its most natural form, so that means organic, unmodified, full-fat versions. The minute we try to make something 'fat-free' we replace the fats with sugars to compensate for flavour and texture.

Salmon, Cherry Tomato and Kale Frittata

Serves 6

The great thing about this frittata is that it is made in a large tray and can supply you with quite a few lunches if you refrigerate or freeze your portions. It's high in protein, packed full of fresh ingredients and is a great use for kale, which is often said to be quite coarse if not cooked until softened.

coconut oil

1 large red onion, finely diced

1 garlic clove, minced

150 g multicoloured cherry tomatoes, halved

1 cup chopped kale leaves, stems removed

1 kg zucchini, grated roughly, water removed (see tip)

6 large eggs

210 g can red salmon in spring water

2 tablespoons chopped flat-leaf parsley

sea salt and ground black pepper

mixed mesclun salad, to serve

avocado oil

lemon juice

1. Preheat oven to 200°C and prepare a large baking dish by greasing well with coconut oil.
2. In a large frying pan, sauté the onion and garlic in a little coconut oil over medium heat until softened and fragrant, then add the cherry tomatoes, kale and zucchini and continue to cook over high heat for about 10 minutes, or until the ingredients are soft and most of the moisture has evaporated. Set aside and allow to cool for 15–20 minutes.
3. Meanwhile, whisk the eggs well in a bowl, then add the salmon and parsley. Gradually add the vegetables, combining well. Don't forget to season the mixture at this stage.
4. Pour the ingredients into the prepared baking dish and bake in the oven for 40–45 minutes, or until cooked through and golden brown on top.
5. Serve with the mixed salad dressed with avocado oil and lemon juice.

TIP: This dish is made with heaps of zucchini, so you need to remove most of the water from them, otherwise your frittata will be too wet. Either squeeze the excess water out with a dishcloth, or place the zucchini in a bowl and cover well with salt to extract the water. Leave for 10–15 minutes. Drain the bowl and pat the zucchini dry before you use it.

Crispy-skin Barramundi with Mango Relish

Serves 4

Barramundi is a fantastically versatile fish – it can be steamed, poached or baked, but what we love is crisping up the skin and serving it with this relish made of fresh fruit and flavoursome herbs. This dish is definitely a crowd-pleaser, with its stunning colour and contrasting textures.

1 red onion, finely diced

1 large mango, diced

1 teaspoon fresh finely grated ginger

juice and zest of 1 lime, zest finely grated

1 Lebanese cucumber, diced

¼ cup chopped fresh coriander

sea salt and ground black pepper

4 barramundi fillets, skin on (about 180 g each)

coconut oil, for frying

mixed greens, to serve

1. Start by whipping up the relish. Combine the onion, mango, ginger, lime juice and zest, cucumber and coriander in a bowl. Season with salt and pepper and set aside.
2. To prepare the barramundi, season the skin really well with salt and pepper. You can score the skin to rub some of this seasoning into the fish itself.
3. Heat a frying pan with the coconut oil, and once the pan is nice and hot, cook the fish, skin side down, for 4–5 minutes, or until skin is crispy and golden and the fish turns slightly opaque. Flip and cook the other side for a few minutes and then set aside to rest. Fish continues cooking once taken off the heat, so be careful not to overcook it.
4. Serve the fish with the mango relish and some mixed greens.

TIP: Where's the sauce? This dish is fantastic when paired with our lime aioli. Check out the recipe on page 126.

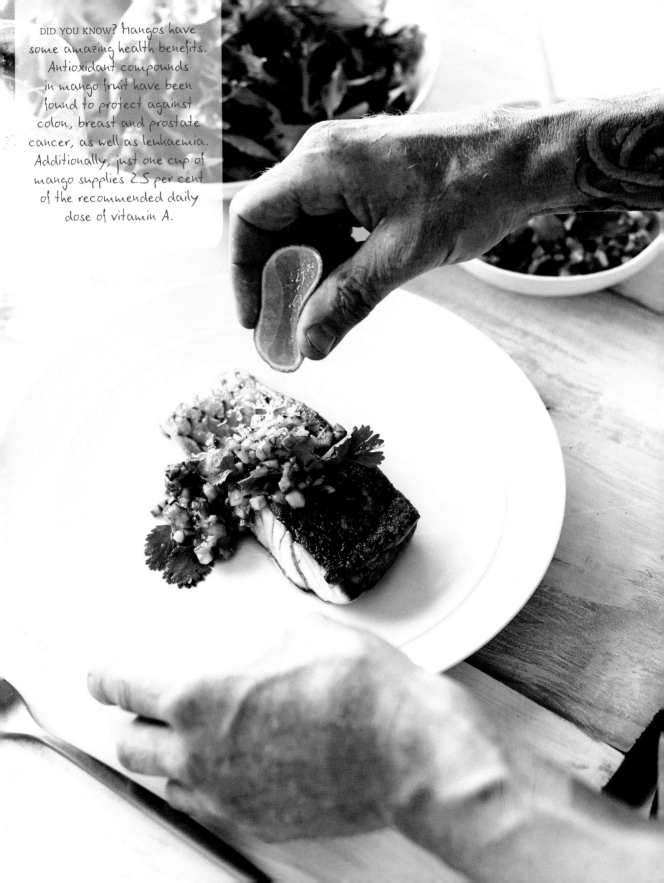

DID YOU KNOW? Mangos have some amazing health benefits. Antioxidant compounds in mango fruit have been found to protect against colon, breast and prostate cancer, as well as leukaemia. Additionally, just one cup of mango supplies 25 per cent of the recommended daily dose of vitamin A.

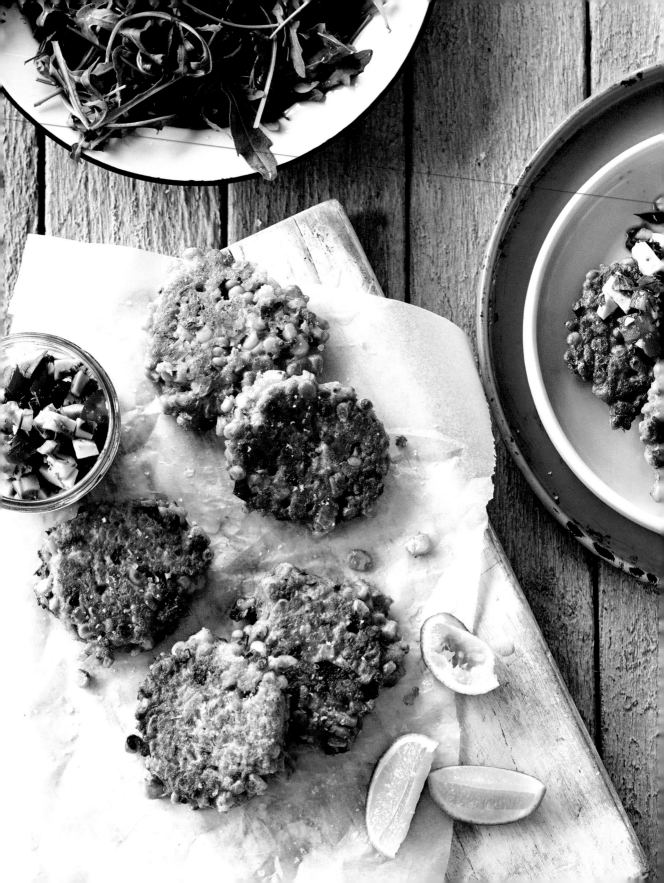

Quinoa and Sweetcorn Fritters with Avocado and Tomato Salsa

Makes 12 fritters

Everyone's familiar with traditional fritters, like pea or corn, but we love adding quinoa into the mix because it really pumps up the protein level and adds such great depth and texture. Perfect for breakfast, lunch or dinner, you cannot go past these delicious fritters for a quick and easy protein hit.

kernels from 3 fresh corn cobs (about 2 cups)

1 cup cooked quinoa (see recipe on page 118), cooled to room temperature

2 tablespoons chopped coriander leaves

2 spring onions, chopped

4 eggs, lightly whisked

¼ cup buckwheat flour

½ teaspoon baking powder

sea salt and ground black pepper

coconut oil, for frying

50 g rocket leaves

Tomato and avocado salsa

1 tomato, diced

2 avocados, diced

½ cup flat-leaf parsley, chopped

¼ red onion, finely chopped

1 tablespoon apple cider vinegar

1 tablespoon lemon juice

1 tablespoon avocado oil

1. Combine the corn kernels, cooked quinoa, coriander, spring onion, eggs, flour, baking powder, salt and pepper in a large bowl. Mix well to form a chunky batter.
2. Fry fritters in the coconut oil, with about ¼ cup of batter forming one fritter. Cook for about 3–4 minutes on each side, until the fritters are a fantastic golden colour.
3. For the tomato and avocado salsa, combine the tomato, avocado, parsley and onion in a bowl and coat well with the combined vinegar, lemon juice and avocado oil.
4. Serve the fritters and salsa on a bed of rocket.

Dinner is the last meal we eat before heading to bed, so it is important we get it right nutritionally. What we consume will be delivered to our body while we sleep and utilised as we rest and recover. We don't want to eat anything too high in sugar or simple carbohydrates, as our bodies don't need as much energy while we're resting.

Dinner is the perfect chance to stock up on protein and vegetables, especially your greens. Structuring your meals like this means dinners are not only good for you, but easy and simple to prepare. When putting your dinner ingredients together, think about what will make you feel healthy and energetic in the morning, while using a variety of colours, flavours and different sources of protein.

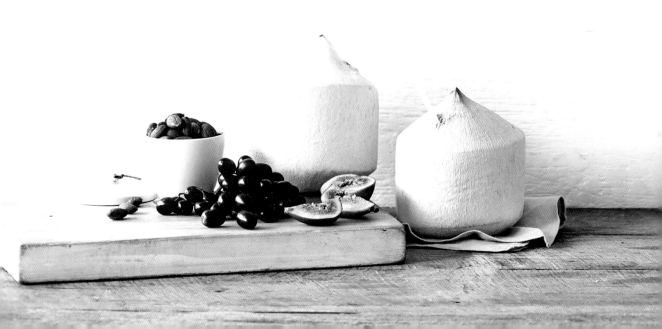

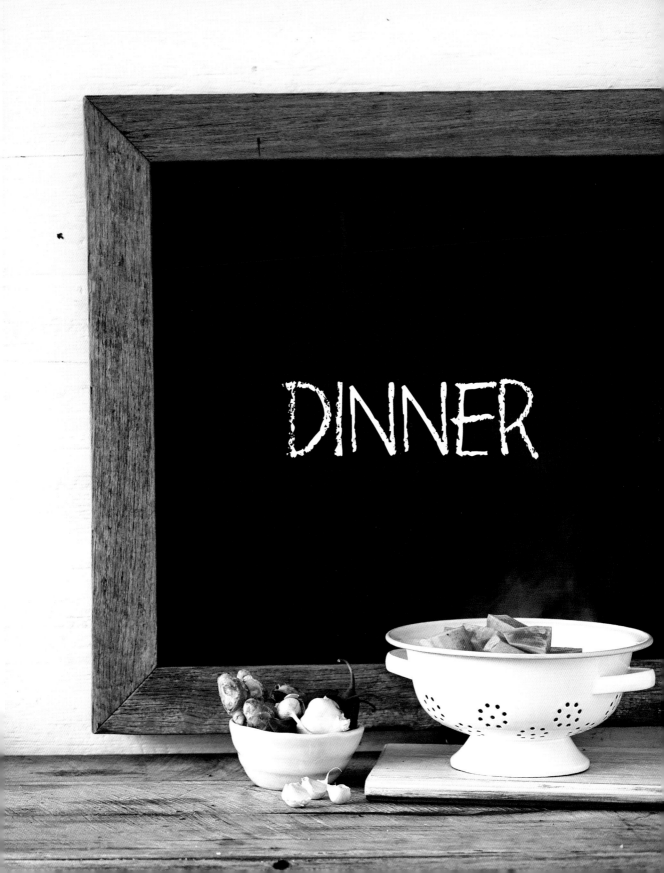

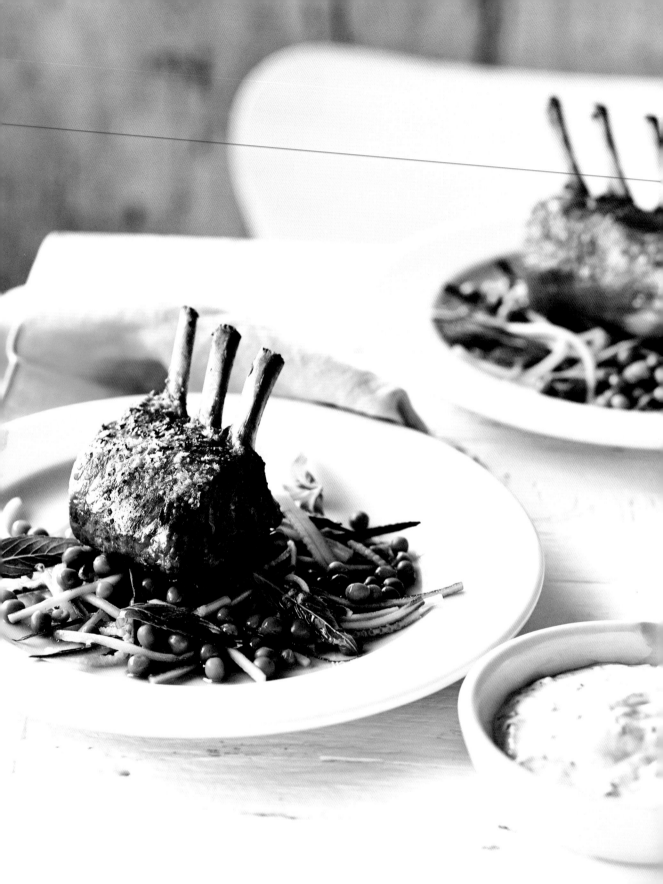

Lamb Cutlets with a Zucchini, Pea and Mint Salad

Serves 4

Nothing says freshness more than this combination of seared lamb cutlets and green salad. Simple, clean and fresh, this meal is a crowd-pleaser and a great way to boost your daily greens intake. The use of mint is awesome, too, because it is often a forgotten herb.

2 zucchini, peeled into fine ribbons

100 g fresh peas

Basic Vinaigrette Dressing (see recipe on page 128)

¼ cup chopped fresh mint leaves

12 lamb cutlets, or 2 six-point lamb racks (600 g in total)

sea salt and cracked pepper

lemon wedges, to serve

Yoghurt Dressing (see recipe on page 128), optional

1. Dress the zucchini ribbons and peas with the vinaigrette and toss the fresh mint in. Mix well and refrigerate until ready to serve.

2. Heat a chargrill pan over high heat and season the cutlets with salt and pepper. Chargrill the cutlets for 2 minutes on each side until medium rare. Transfer to a plate and cover with foil to rest for 5 minutes. If using lamb racks, bake at 200°C for 12 minutes and, once rested, slice each rack in half.

3. Serve with the salad and lemon wedges. Our yoghurt dressing also goes really well with this dish.

TIP: Try cooking this one on the barbecue grill. Not only does meat taste even better when cooked over an open flame, but you get the char marks from the grill, making it look amazing!

Adobo Roast Chicken

Serves 4

Welcome to our take on a true taste of Mexico! The adobo spice mixture is a traditional Mexican spice rub that can be used on numerous cuts of meat. We love basting our roast chicken with it, and pairing it with a zesty red cabbage salad and a traditional chimichurri sauce. It's like a deconstructed taco on your plate, and with the addition of some fresh chilli (if you're brave), it can rock your socks off.

1 tablespoon chilli powder

2 teaspoons sea salt

2 teaspoons paprika

2 teaspoons sugar

1 teaspoon onion powder

½ teaspoon garlic powder

½ teaspoon cayenne

½ teaspoon ground cumin

1.8 kg whole organic chicken

2 tablespoon coconut oil, melted

2 lemons

Red Cabbage and Lime Slaw
  (see recipe on page 122)

Chimichurri (see recipe on
  page 129)

1. Preheat oven to 220°C and lightly grease a roasting pan.
2. Combine the chilli powder, salt, paprika, sugar, onion powder, garlic powder, cayenne and cumin together to make the adobo.
3. Coat the chicken well with the coconut oil and adobo mix, then drizzle with the juice of one lemon.
4. Next, pierce a few holes into the remaining lemon with a knife and stuff it in the cavity of the chicken.
5. Place a wire rack in the roasting pan and put the chicken on top. Whack it in the oven and roast for 60–80 minutes, or until the juices run clear when a chicken thigh is pierced with a skewer. (You can make the slaw and chimichurri sauce while the chicken is roasting, if you haven't prepared them in advance.)
6. Remove the chicken from the oven and allow to stand, covered, for 10 minutes. Carve and serve with the slaw and chimichurri.

VARIATION: Different cuts of chicken really work with this dish. Try marinating some chicken thighs in the adobo mix and then chargrilling them on the barbecue.

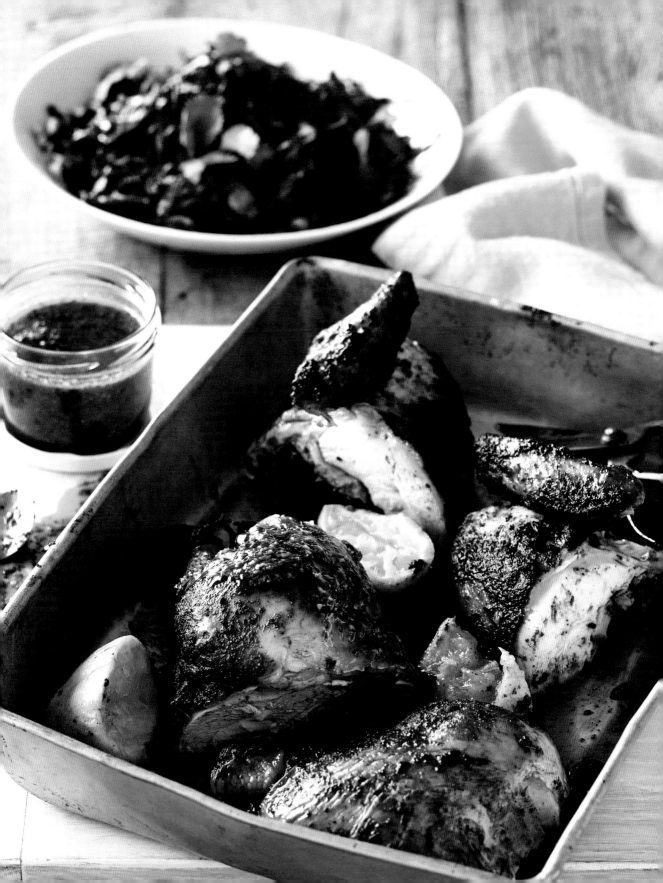

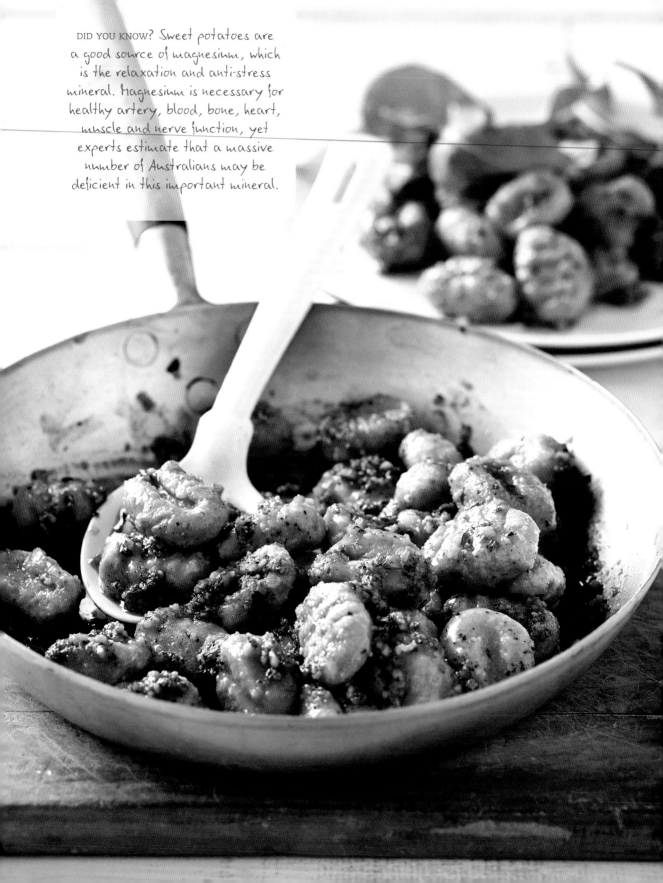

DID YOU KNOW? Sweet potatoes are a good source of magnesium, which is the relaxation and anti-stress mineral. Magnesium is necessary for healthy artery, blood, bone, heart, muscle and nerve function, yet experts estimate that a massive number of Australians may be deficient in this important mineral.

Sweet Potato Gnocchi

Serves 4

Craving pasta but don't want to fill up on starchy foods like white potatoes and regular wheat flour? Try our fresh sweet potato gnocchi for a filling and healthy pasta dish. The great thing about this recipe is that everything is made from scratch. Try serving it with our Pounded Walnut Sauce – it's a wicked one for vegetarians (see recipe on page 127).

750 g small orange sweet potato, unpeeled

500 g small desiree potatoes, unpeeled

sea salt and ground black pepper

1 egg yolk

2 cups fine quinoa flour

butter, for frying

avocado oil, for frying

pasta sauce, to serve

fresh herbs, to garnish

1. Steam the potato and sweet potato, whole and unpeeled, for about 45 minutes. Once they are tender, remove from the steamer and let them cool a little. Remove the skins and mash the flesh in a bowl until it is smooth. Season with salt and pepper and set aside.

2. Once the potato mash has cooled completely, add the egg yolk and quinoa flour. Stir until the dough is firm, then turn out onto a floured surface. Knead until smooth. (If the dough is too sticky, you may need to add more quinoa flour).

3. Divide the dough into 6 portions and roll each portion into a log about 40 cm long. Lightly flour a knife and cut the log into 2 cm pieces. Do this with each of the 6 dough portions. Then, roll each 2 cm piece of dough into a little ball. To make the grooves that you see in gnocchi, press with a floured fork.

4. Cook gnocchi in a gently simmering pot of water until they float to the top. Lift out with a slotted spoon.

5. Meanwhile, heat a frying pan over medium heat, add butter and avocado oil and, once the gnocchi has cooled, pan-fry on each side until lightly browned.

6. Serve with your favourite pasta sauce, or try the Pounded Walnut Sauce on page 127. Top with a sprinkling of fresh herbs.

TIP: When making gnocchi, you need to be intuitive. If you find your dough is looking a little too wet, add more flour, and add water if it's looking a little dry. The key to the best fresh pasta is being able to adapt to the process.

Pecan-crusted Tuna

Serves 4

We love this meal because it really makes the most of delicious fresh tuna. It's the type of seafood that only needs to be seared briefly and eaten rare to enjoy maximum flavour. Serve it with our Superfood Pink Grapefruit and Black Quinoa Salad (see page 119) for a double hit of protein.

1 tablespoon coconut oil, plus extra for frying

1 tablespoon unsalted butter

1 tablespoon chopped flat-leaf parsley

1 large dried chilli, crumbled

800 g sashimi-grade tuna

150 g pecans, crushed and roasted

sea salt and ground black pepper

1. Heat the coconut oil, butter, parsley and chilli in a small saucepan, only until the oil and butter have melted together. Reserve the mixture and allow to cool slightly.

2. Roll the tuna in the oil mixture and then coat with the crushed roasted pecans.

3. Heat a large frying pan to very hot and pan-fry the tuna till seared on all sides. Let it rest before serving to allow the butter coating to cool and set, holding the pecans in place. Thinly slice the tuna and season before serving.

TIP: When searing your tuna, make sure the pan is nice and hot. Protein can stew if the pan isn't hot enough. You want the tuna to sizzle upon touching so that it seals well and creates good colour and caramelisation.

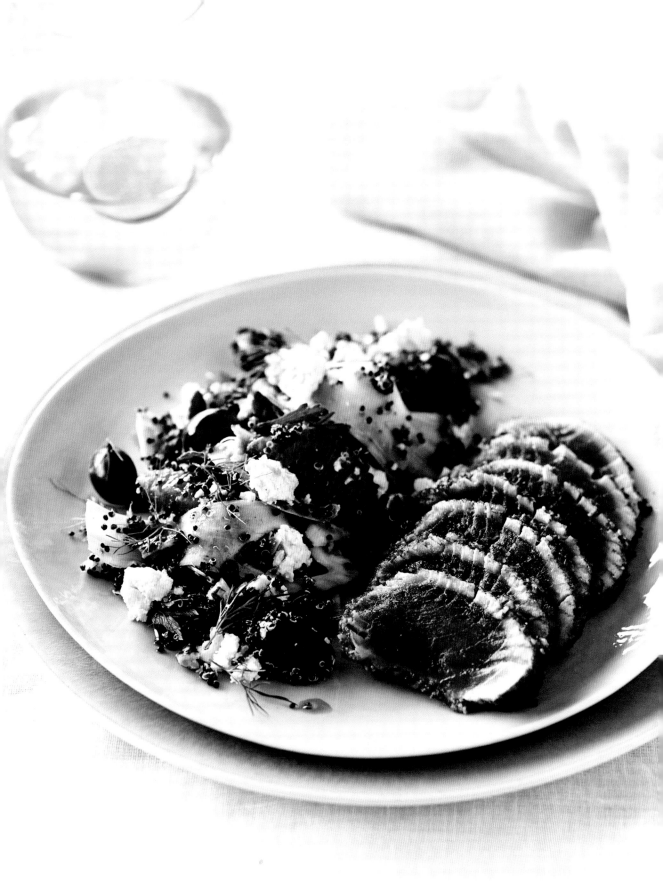

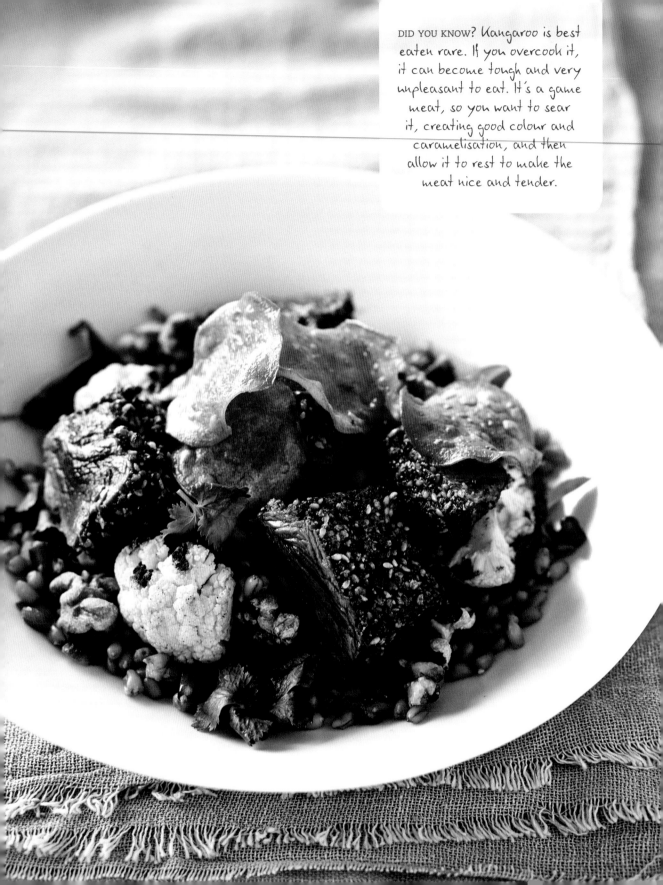

DID YOU KNOW? Kangaroo is best eaten rare. If you overcook it, it can become tough and very unpleasant to eat. It's a game meat, so you want to sear it, creating good colour and caramelisation, and then allow it to rest to make the meat nice and tender.

Dukkah Kangaroo

Serves 4

Kangaroo is one of our favourite meats. Not only is it extremely high in protein, low in fat and pumped full of iron, it is a sustainable choice due to healthy farming practices. When cooking kangaroo, it is simply a case of searing it in a hot pan so that the meat stays rare and tender – game meats, like roo, have to be kept nice and pink to be enjoyed to the fullest.

½ cup pine nuts

½ cup coriander seeds

¾ cup sesame seeds

½ teaspoon ground cumin

½ teaspoon sea salt

½ teaspoon chilli powder

½ teaspoon baharat (white and black pepper, cinnamon, cloves and nutmeg)

800 g kangaroo fillets

coconut oil, for frying

Freekeh, Roast Cauliflower and Pomegranate Salad, to serve (see recipe on page 123)

Sweet Potato Discs, to garnish (see recipe on page 126)

1. Heat a large frying pan over medium-high heat and toast the pine nuts and coriander seeds (without any oil) until the mix has started to colour. Add the sesame seeds and continue to toast until golden brown. Be careful not to let them burn! Cool completely, then pour the mixture into a food processor.
2. Add the cumin, baharat mix, chilli powder and salt. Blend together to make the dukkah, and tip the mix onto a plate.
3. Roll the kangaroo fillets in the dukkah, then pan-sear in coconut oil over high heat for about 2 minutes on each side, until brown, and then let rest for 5 minutes. Slice for serving, and serve with the salad and sweet potato discs.

TIP: Try this dish with our lime aioli (see recipe on page 126). Although not a traditional pairing, we love smearing our kangaroo through it to just enhance the flavours.

Crispy-skin Ocean Trout with Pea Puree

Serves 4

Ocean trout is a great fish to eat in place of salmon. It's often tempting to avoid white fish, as it can be slightly harder to cook than red fish, but ocean trout is super easy to cook. It's such a fresh, summery dish that really lends itself to be served alongside a crisp green salad (try our Fennel and Zucchini Salad).

1½ cups frozen peas

15 g unsalted butter

2 teaspoons coconut oil, for
  frying, plus 1 tablespoon for fish

2 eschalots, peeled and chopped

¾ cup chicken stock

1 sprig of chervil

1 tablespoon lemon juice

sea salt and ground black pepper

4 × 180 gram ocean trout fillets

Fennel and Zucchini Salad,
  to serve (see recipe on page 122)

1. Spread the peas on a tray and allow them to thaw for 10 minutes.
2. Place a large frying pan over medium heat, add the coconut oil and half the butter, then add the eschalots and sauté until soft.
3. In another small saucepan, bring the chicken stock to the boil.
4. Add the peas to the eschalots along with the chervil and lemon juice. Pour the hot chicken stock over the peas and quickly bring up to the boil, then remove from the heat and allow to cool slightly.
5. Pour the pea mixture into a blender and process until fine. Adjust seasoning accordingly.
6. Score the skin of the ocean trout, season with salt and brush with a little coconut oil. Heat a frying pan over high heat, add the remaining coconut oil and butter and cook the fish, skin side down, until crispy. Flip once, simply sealing the top.
7. Serve the trout with the pea puree and a fennel and zucchini salad on the side. Or, to pump up the carbs, serve with some roasted sweet potato.

VARIATION: Not a fan of ocean trout? You could try another oily fish like salmon or rainbow trout, or even a beautiful white fish like blue-eye trevalla or barramundi.

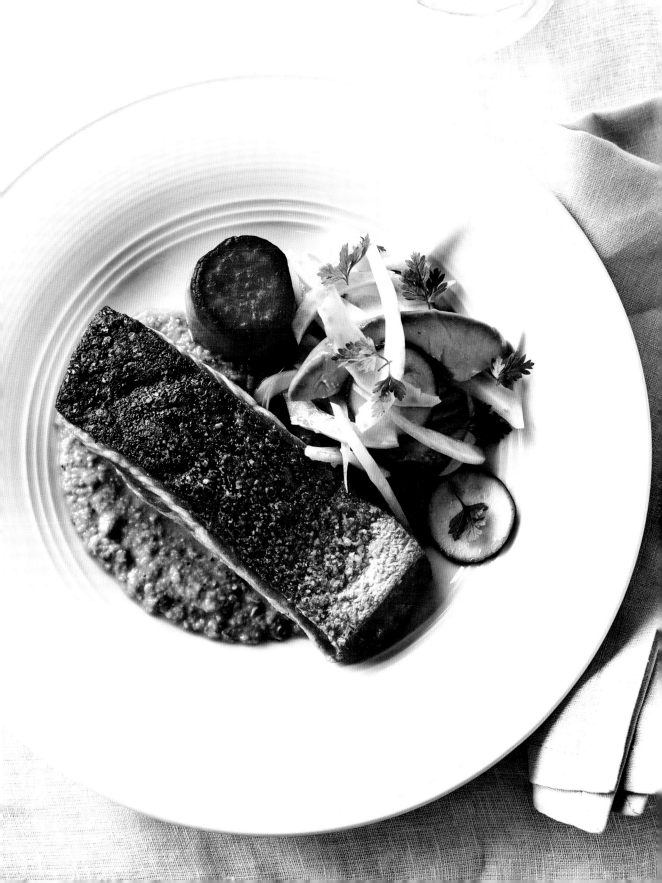

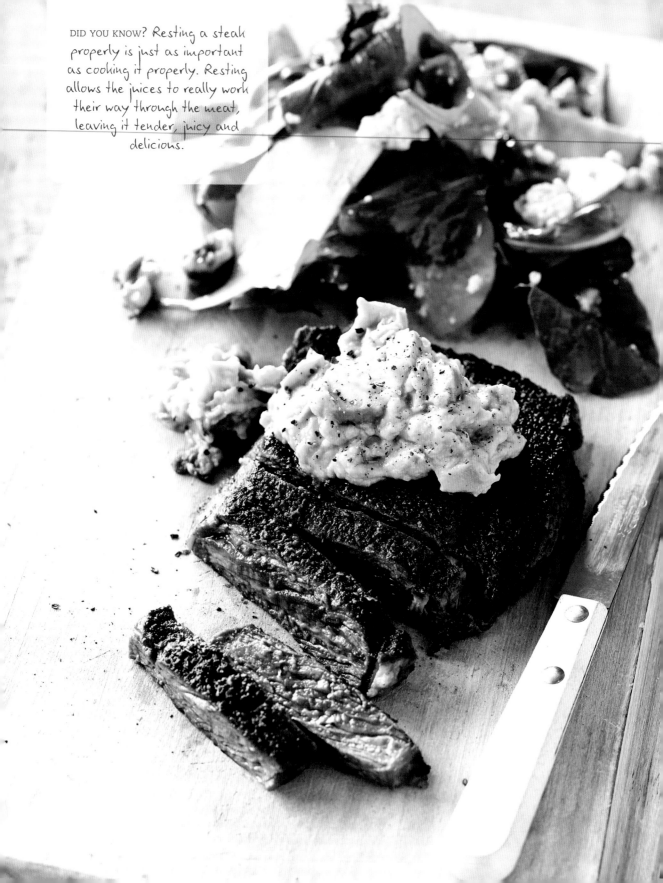

DID YOU KNOW? Resting a steak properly is just as important as cooking it properly. Resting allows the juices to really work their way through the meat, leaving it tender, juicy and delicious.

Chilli Salt Scotch Fillet with Avocado and a Pear and Rocket Salad

Serves 4

Sometimes the end of the day calls for a big hunk of meat, and what fits the bill better than our famous Chilli Salt Scotch Fillet? Simple to prepare but phenomenal to eat when paired with a pear and rocket salad, this one is sure to please.

3 garlic cloves

¼ teaspoon dried chilli flakes

1 teaspoon dried oregano

sea salt flakes

1 tablespoon melted coconut oil, for coating, plus extra for frying

4 × 200–220 gram scotch fillets

4 packed cups baby rocket (about 80 g)

1 pear, finely sliced lengthways

¼ cup walnuts, toasted

⅓ cup goat's feta, crumbled (optional)

Basic Vinaigrette Dressing (see recipe on page 128)

2 avocados

2 tablespoons freshly squeezed lemon juice

1 teaspoon finely chopped flat-leaf parsley

1 teaspoon finely chopped fresh chives

ground black pepper

1. Roughly chop one garlic clove. Using a mortar and pestle, pound the chopped garlic, chilli flakes, oregano, 2 teaspoons of sea salt and the coconut oil to make a paste. Rub the paste over each scotch fillet steak, coating all sides.

2. Heat some more coconut oil in a large heavy-based frying pan over high heat. Add the steaks and cook for about 3 minutes each side for medium-rare. Transfer the steaks to a warm plate and allow to rest for 5 minutes.

3. Mix the rocket, pear, walnuts and feta together well, dress with the vinaigrette and set aside.

4. Mince the two remaining garlic cloves, then peel and pit the avocados. Dice half of one of the avocados and set aside. In a bowl, combine the remaining avocado flesh with the minced garlic, lemon juice, parsley, chives and a few pinches of salt and pepper. Blitz in a blender and pulse until combined. Once done, stir in the chopped avocado to give it texture.

5. Serve the steak with a generous dollop of avocado on top and the rocket salad on the side.

VARIATION: Our other favourite cut of meat to do this way is the rib eye. No matter what cut of beef you go with, make sure you keep it tasting great by cooking it carefully and allowing it to rest.

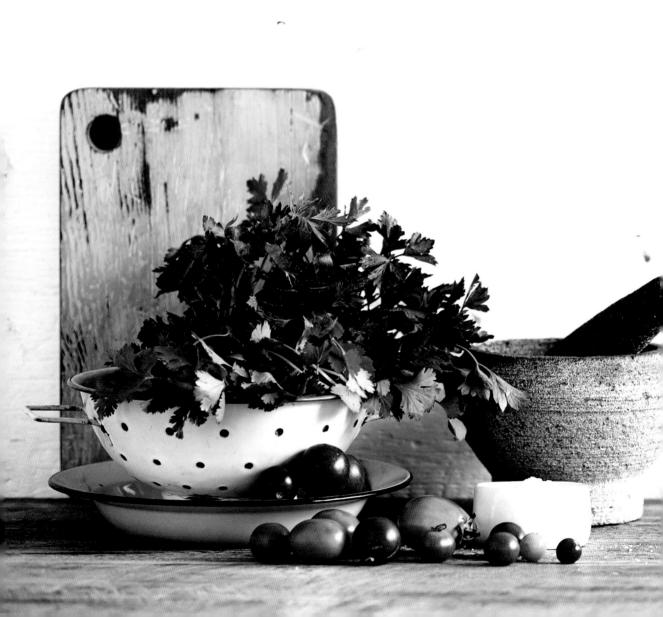

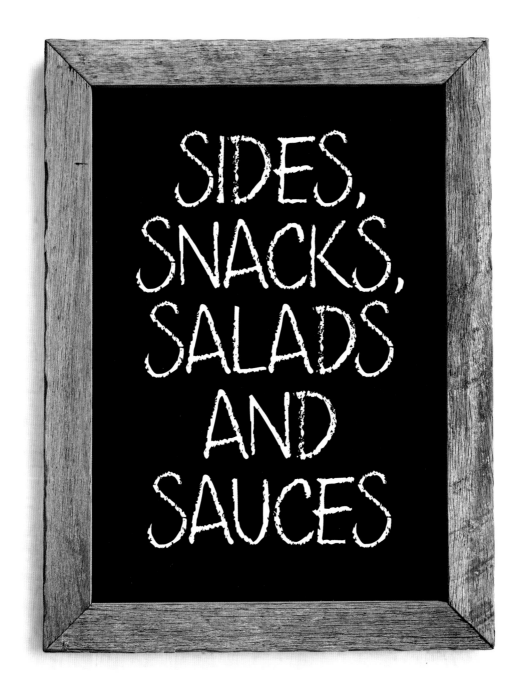

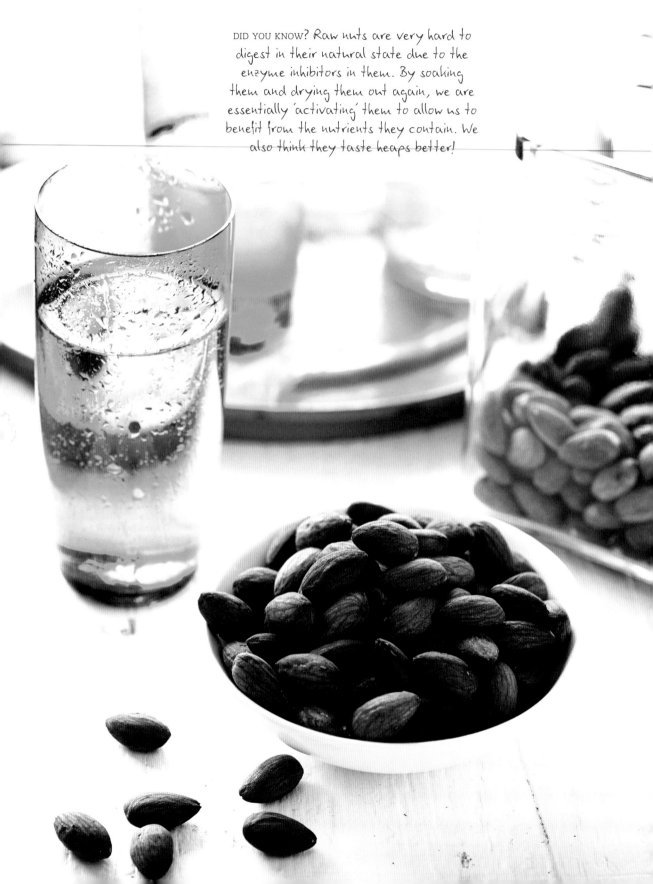

DID YOU KNOW? Raw nuts are very hard to digest in their natural state due to the enzyme inhibitors in them. By soaking them and drying them out again, we are essentially 'activating' them to allow us to benefit from the nutrients they contain. We also think they taste heaps better!

Activated Almonds

Makes 1 kilo

It's time to activate your nuts! We've mentioned these infamous nuts a few times, especially in our breakfast section. And guess what, you can save your cash and make them yourself. They store well in the freezer, so you can make a big batch of them and have them ready to go. This recipe is for activated almonds, but you can try doing this with any non-oily nut or seed, like pecans or walnuts.

1 kg almonds

pinch of sea salt

1. Soak the almonds overnight in a saucepan of salted water, keeping the lid on.
2. Drain well, then spread the nuts out on an oven tray and dry them in the oven for no less than 12 hours with your oven set at its lowest temperature. Less than 65°C is ideal.
3. Let them cool, and then store them in a sealed container in the fridge.

VARIATION: Try making an activated mix. Combine almonds, pepitas and pecans together and follow the recipe above, creating a great snack mix to eat at work or on the run.

Cacao-nut Crunch Clusters

Makes 26

These are a delicious treat – both decadent and nutritious. They are packed full of raw nuts, providing you with a high-protein snack that will keep you feeling full. The other great thing about these nut clusters is how simple they are to make.

2 tablespoons coconut oil

⅓ cup honey

½ cup peanut or almond butter

1 teaspoon vanilla extract

2 cups shredded coconut

1 tablespoon chia seeds

¼ cup cacao powder

¼ cup chopped walnuts

¼ cup toasted slivered almonds

1. In a large saucepan, melt the coconut oil over very low heat. Add the honey and nut butter and gently stir to combine, then add the remaining ingredients and stir them through.
2. Using a spoon, scoop tablespoonfuls of the mixture onto a baking tray or large plates. Store some in the fridge to set, ready for eating once firm, and put any extras in the freezer for a later date.

NOTE: These actually provide a terrific pre-exercise energy hit. And because the nut clusters are only small, you won't feel too full to train.

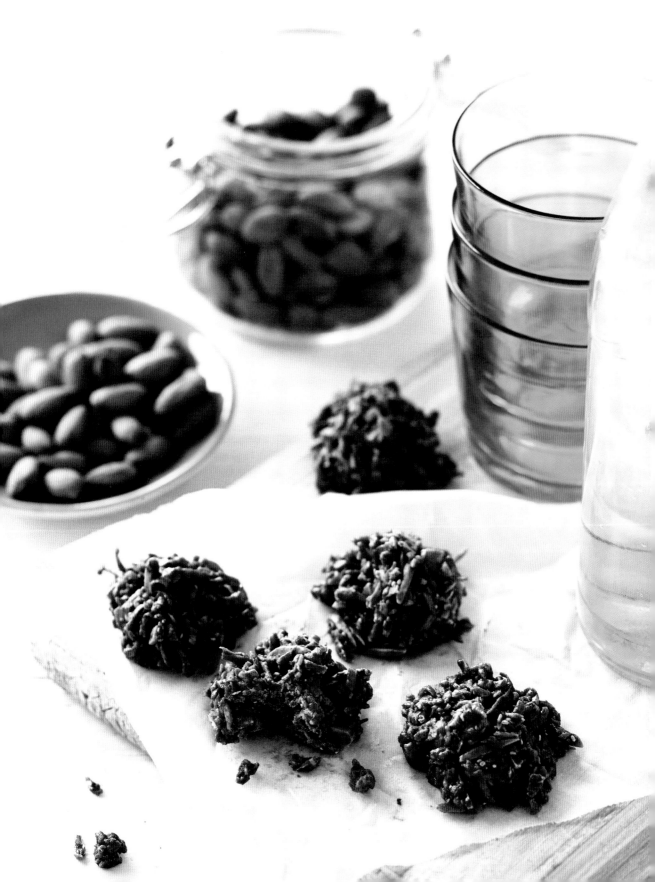

The Perfect Quinoa

Makes 3 cups cooked quinoa

Pronounced keen-wah, quinoa is an ancient seed made famous by the Inca warriors, who were the first to discover its phenomenal health benefits. It's a fantastic replacement for rice or pasta and is free of gluten and wheat. It's easy to cook, freezes forever and can be used for breakfast, lunch and dinner. Quinoa certainly deserves its superfood bragging rights – it's a high-energy food containing all eight amino acids, making it a complete protein. It transforms from a crunchy seed to a fluffy, slightly coiled sprout in mere minutes – pretty cool!

good pinch of sea salt

1 cup uncooked quinoa, rinsed

1. Bring 1½ cups of salted water up to the boil, then add the quinoa.
2. Bring back to the boil (which won't take long at all), then immediately reduce to the lowest heat possible and simmer very gently, with the lid on, for 15 minutes. Don't stir it, touch it or move it – I know you will be tempted to, but just trust us here.
3. Remove the pot from the heat and set aside, with the lid still on, for about 5 minutes.
4. And that's it. All you have to do now is run a fork through the quinoa to fluff it up before serving. Perfect!

TIP: Quinoa has to be rinsed well before cooking. It has a naturally occurring bitter coating called saponin, which is mildly toxic. Rinsing removes the saponin. Once there is no more soapy residue, you know you've washed it all off.

Superfood Pink Grapefruit and Black Quinoa Salad

Serves 4 as a side dish

The great thing about this super fresh and healthy salad is the diverse range of ingredients. The combination of the quinoa, the citrus of the grapefruit, the creaminess of the feta and the sweetness of the grapes is amazing. It goes really well with our Pecan-crusted Tuna (see recipe on page 104).

40 g pecans

1 cup uncooked black quinoa

1 pink grapefruit

1 fennel bulb, halved lengthwise, sliced paper thin, reserve the fronds

1 cup seedless red grapes

70 g goat's feta cheese, crumbled (optional)

2 tablespoons chopped flat-leaf parsley

1 tablespoon chopped chives

1 tablespoon chopped dill

Basic Vinaigrette Dressing (see page 128)

1. Preheat the oven to 180°C and line a tray with baking paper.
2. Toast the pecans in the oven for 8–10 minutes, until they are fragrant and even light brown. Allow to cool, then chop them roughly and set aside.
3. Cook the black quinoa and check constantly. (For tips on cooking perfect quinoa every time, see opposite.)
4. Peel the pink grapefruit and remove the pith. Cut into segments, halve and set aside until ready to serve.
5. In a large mixing bowl, combine the pecans, quinoa, pink grapefruit, fennel, grapes and feta. Add the dressing and fresh herbs and toss very gently. Serve topped with a little parsley and reserved fennel fronds.

VARIATION: The citrus and pecans in this dish make it a delicious accompaniment to crispy-skin duck. If you're a fan of duck, cook up a fillet, get the skin nice and crisp, then slice the duck and toss it through the finished salad.

Broccolini with Almonds and Fresh Chilli

Serves 4 as a side dish

Looking for a side dish to pump up your daily vegetable intake? Try this beautiful and simple broccolini dish. Easy to prepare and rich in flavour, it's great to serve up as a share plate at a dinner party.

1 bunch broccolini

1 tablespoon coconut oil

1 small garlic clove, sliced

1 long red chilli, finely chopped

50 g slivered almonds, toasted

a pinch of lemon zest

sea salt and ground black pepper

1. Blanch the broccolini in a pot of boiling water, remove from the water when still crisp, pat dry with a tea towel and set aside.

2. Heat a large frying pan with coconut oil, add the garlic and chilli and sauté until tender and slightly golden. Now add the blanched broccolini and toss well to combine.

3. Remove from the heat, sprinkle with the toasted almonds and lemon zest, and season to taste.

VARIATION: Like your chilli hot? Swap the long red chilli for a short bullet chilli or two, to really give your broccolini a hit.

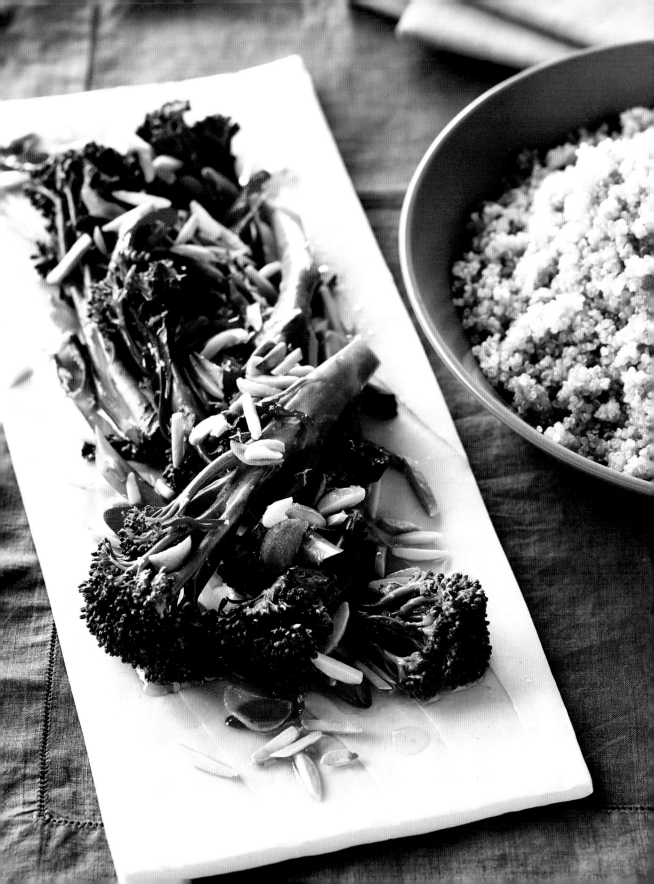

Red Cabbage and Lime Slaw

Serves 4 as a side dish

We don't think red cabbage is used enough. It's an amazing source of vitamin C that can help maintain beautiful skin and delay the ageing process. Try this with our Adobo Roast Chicken (see recipe on page 100).

¼ red cabbage, thinly sliced

1 red apple, cored and sliced into very thin discs

½ bunch fresh coriander, chopped

2 tablespoons apple cider vinegar

2 tablespoons avocado oil

1 tablespoon rice malt syrup

1 tablespoon lime juice

1. In a large bowl, combine the cabbage and apple. Add the coriander and mix well.
2. In another bowl, whisk together the vinegar, lime juice, avocado oil and rice malt syrup.
3. Pour the dressing over the salad and coat well. The longer you let the cabbage sit in the dressing, the more it will soften, which is a really nice result.

Fennel and Zucchini Salad

Serves 4 as a side dish

This salad goes especially well with fish, and complements our Crispy-skin Ocean Trout with Pea Puree beautifully (see recipe on page 108).

2 fennel bulbs

2 zucchini, cut into thin discs

1 avocado, cut into small segments and thinly sliced

1. Finely slice or julienne the fennel bulbs and mix with the zucchini discs and avocado segments.
2. Toss the salad gently with Basic Vinaigrette Dressing (see recipe on page 128) to coat well.

Freekeh, Roast Cauliflower and Pomegranate Salad

Serves 4 as a side dish

This salad is a taste of the Middle East. It uses the ancient grain freekeh, which is becoming quite trendy at restaurants these days as an alternative to rice. Although freekeh isn't paleo, it's low carb, low GI and higher in protein, vitamins and minerals than other grains – and it tastes fantastic, too. Try it with our Dukkah Kangaroo (see recipe on page 107).

1½ cups wholegrain freekeh

2 tablespoons coconut oil

1 brown onion, finely chopped

¼ cup buckwheat or fine quinoa flour

1 teaspoon ground cumin

1 teaspoon ground coriander

½ cauliflower (about 1 kg, untrimmed), broken into small florets

seeds of 1 pomegranate

1 cup walnuts, toasted

⅓ cup mint (small whole leaves)

⅓ cup coriander (small whole leaves)

⅓ cup basil (small whole leaves)

2 tablespoons avocado oil

2 tablespoons pomegranate molasses

1. Soak the freekeh in cold water for 5 minutes, then drain.
2. Heat one tablespoon of the coconut oil in a medium saucepan and sauté the onion until softened. Add the freekeh, then 1 litre of water, and simmer for 45 minutes or until the water has been absorbed and the freekeh is tender.
3. Meanwhile, mix the flour, cumin and coriander in a large bowl. Toss the cauliflower in the spiced flour to coat.
4. Heat the remaining coconut oil in a large, deep frying pan. Add the spice-dusted cauliflower and fry over medium-low heat for 10 minutes, or until the cauliflower is soft and golden. Add a little extra oil if required.
5. Toss the cauliflower with the freekeh, pomegranate seeds, toasted walnuts and fresh herbs. Drizzle with avocado oil and pomegranate molasses, and serve.

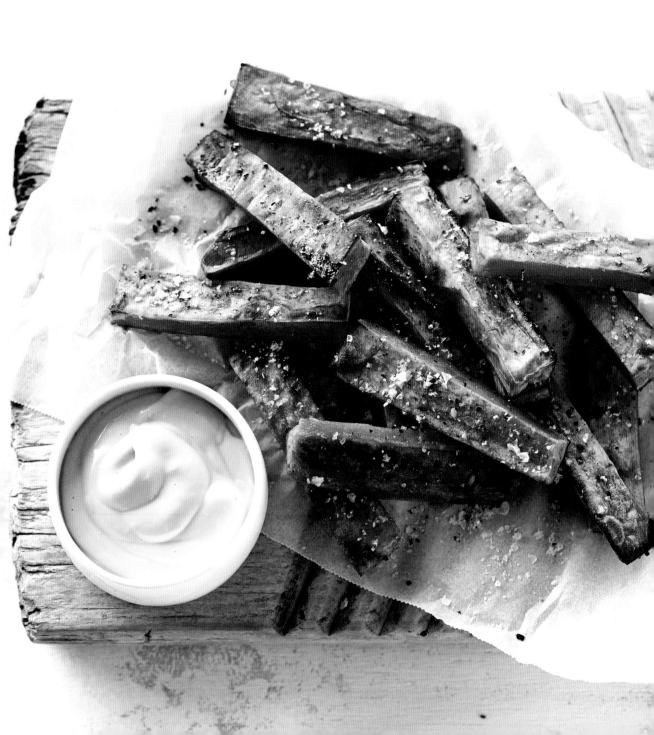

Sweet Potato Fries

Serves 4

Sometimes you just need a great-tasting snack to fill that afternoon void, or perhaps the perfect crunchy addition to your lunch or dinner. Look no further than our crunchy sweet potato fries.

2 large sweet potatoes

1 tablespoon coconut oil, melted

sea salt and ground black pepper

Lime Aioli (see recipe on
  page 126)

1. Preheat oven to 220°C and then prep the potato. We like to leave the skin on because that's where so many of the nutrients are. If you wash your potato, make sure you dry it really, really well. You don't want any moisture, after all – you want crunchy fries.

2. Cut the sweet potatoes in half, because they're normally very large. Now take half a potato and slice it longways, making each slice about 2 cm thick. Then cut these larger slices into long fries about 1.5 cm thick. Repeat this with the remaining potato halves.

3. Place the prepared fries on a large baking tray and drizzle with coconut oil, then season with a generous amount of salt and pepper. Bake in the oven for 30–45 minutes, turning the chips halfway through the cooking time. Remove from the oven, add more salt and pepper if need be, then serve with our lime aioli.

TIP: Try not to open the oven more than once while the fries are baking. You need the oven to be really hot to get them as crisp as possible. As tempting as it is to keep opening the oven door, just let them bake away!

Lime Aioli

Makes ½ cup

This is our favourite addition to just about any recipe. It's fresh, zesty and creamy all at the same time, and we can't get enough of it, particularly with meat dishes, but it's good with vegies too. Make some of our amazing sweet potato fries and try whipping up this aioli to go with it. The combination of the sweetness of the potato and the zesty aioli is yum.

2 egg yolks

1 teaspoon Dijon mustard

125 ml avocado oil (plus a little extra, if needed)

¼ garlic clove, minced

zest of 1 lime

1 teaspoon lime juice

1. Combine the egg yolks with the Dijon mustard in a small bowl.
2. While whisking very fast, slowly and gradually pour in the avocado oil, making sure the mixture doesn't split.
3. Once the mixture is thick and creamy, add the garlic, lime juice and lime zest and stir through.

Sweet Potato Discs

Makes 8 discs

This crispy side works really well with our Dukkah Kangaroo (page 107).

2 sweet potatoes (about 600 g)

coconut oil

1 tablespoon butter

sea salt and ground black pepper

1. Using a peeler, finely slice the sweet potatoes.
2. Shallow fry in coconut oil and butter in a hot frying pan until golden and crispy. Season to taste.

Pounded Walnut Sauce

Serves 4

We recommend pairing this delicious sauce with our Sweet Potato Gnocchi (page 103), but it also goes beautifully with all pasta options. Its texture is really similar to a pesto, and with the combination of crushed walnuts and vibrant herbs, it has the flavour to match. We don't eat a lot of dairy, so we make it without the pecorino, but you can add it in for extra richness and flavour.

1 cup walnuts

1 clove garlic

⅔ cup avocado oil

4 tablespoons marjoram, chopped

2 tablespoons parsley, chopped

2 tablespoons basil leaves,
  chopped

small handful of baby rocket
  leaves

½ cup pecorino, finely grated
  (optional)

sea salt and cracked black pepper

cooked pasta, to serve

1. Place the walnuts on a lined baking tray and bake them in a preheated 180°C oven for about 10 minutes or until golden. Bring them out of the oven, wrap them in a clean tea towel and rub off their skins. Set aside.

2. Place the garlic and ½ teaspoon of sea salt in a mortar and pestle, and pound to a fine paste. Add the walnuts and continue pounding.

3. Transfer the nut paste to a bowl and stir in the avocado oil, then add most of the herbs and rocket leaves (keep a few pinches to use as a garnish). Stir in the pecorino, if you're using it, and adjust the seasoning to taste.

4. Toss the sauce with the pasta, and serve topped with the extra herbs.

VARIATION: Want to pump up your protein? How about topping your pasta with some crisp prosciutto? Simply place strips of prosciutto on an oven tray and bake on a high heat for 2–3 minutes until crisp, then break up and sprinkle over the top for a meaty hit and added crunch.

Yoghurt Dressing

Remember to choose full-fat Greek yoghurt to avoid added sugar. Lots of low-fat products on the market actually contain excessive amounts of added sugar to improve the taste after the fat has been removed. Try this dressing with our Lamb Cutlets (page 99).

⅔ cup plain Greek yoghurt

⅓ fresh chilli, stemmed, seeded and minced

¼ cup fresh mint leaves

¼ cup fresh coriander leaves

1½ tablespoons honey or rice malt syrup

⅓ teaspoon ground cumin, toasted

a pinch of sea salt

1. Place all ingredients into a food processor and mix until combined. Add a little water, if it is too thick.
2. Add salt to taste.

Basic Vinaigrette Dressing

We use this dressing on all kinds of salads. Simple but tasty.

2 tablespoons apple cider vinegar

1 garlic clove, minced

1 teaspoon rice malt syrup or maple syrup

½ cup avocado oil

1. In a small bowl, add the ingredients in the order listed.
2. Whisk to combine.

Chimichurri

This deliciously zingy sauce works well with our Adobo Roast Chicken (page 100).

1 bunch flat leaf parsley

6 cloves of garlic, smashed

½ cup avocado oil

¼ cup apple cider vinegar

juice of half a lemon

½ red onion, diced

sea salt and black pepper

1. Mix all the ingredients, except the seasonings, in a food processor, adding slightly more avocado oil for a wetter sauce if you desire.

2. Add salt and pepper to taste.

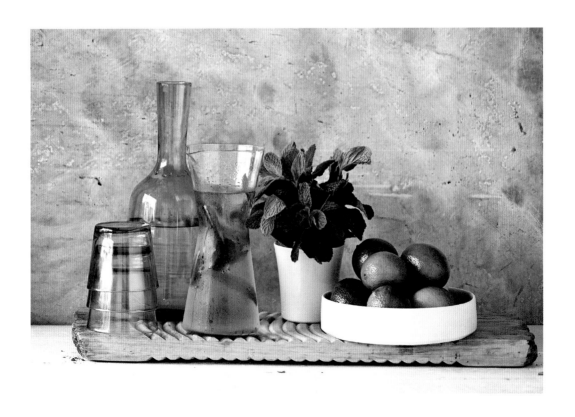

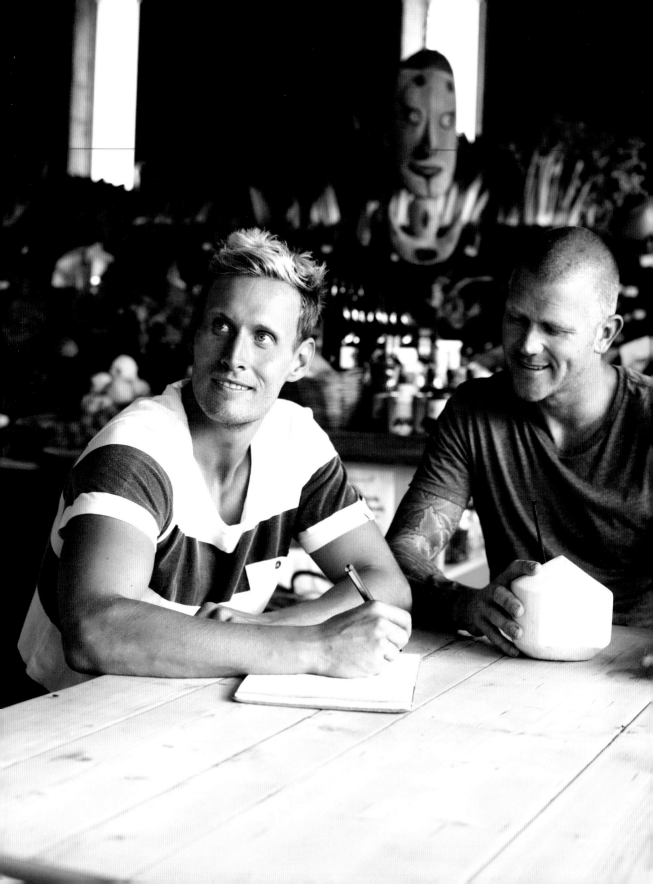

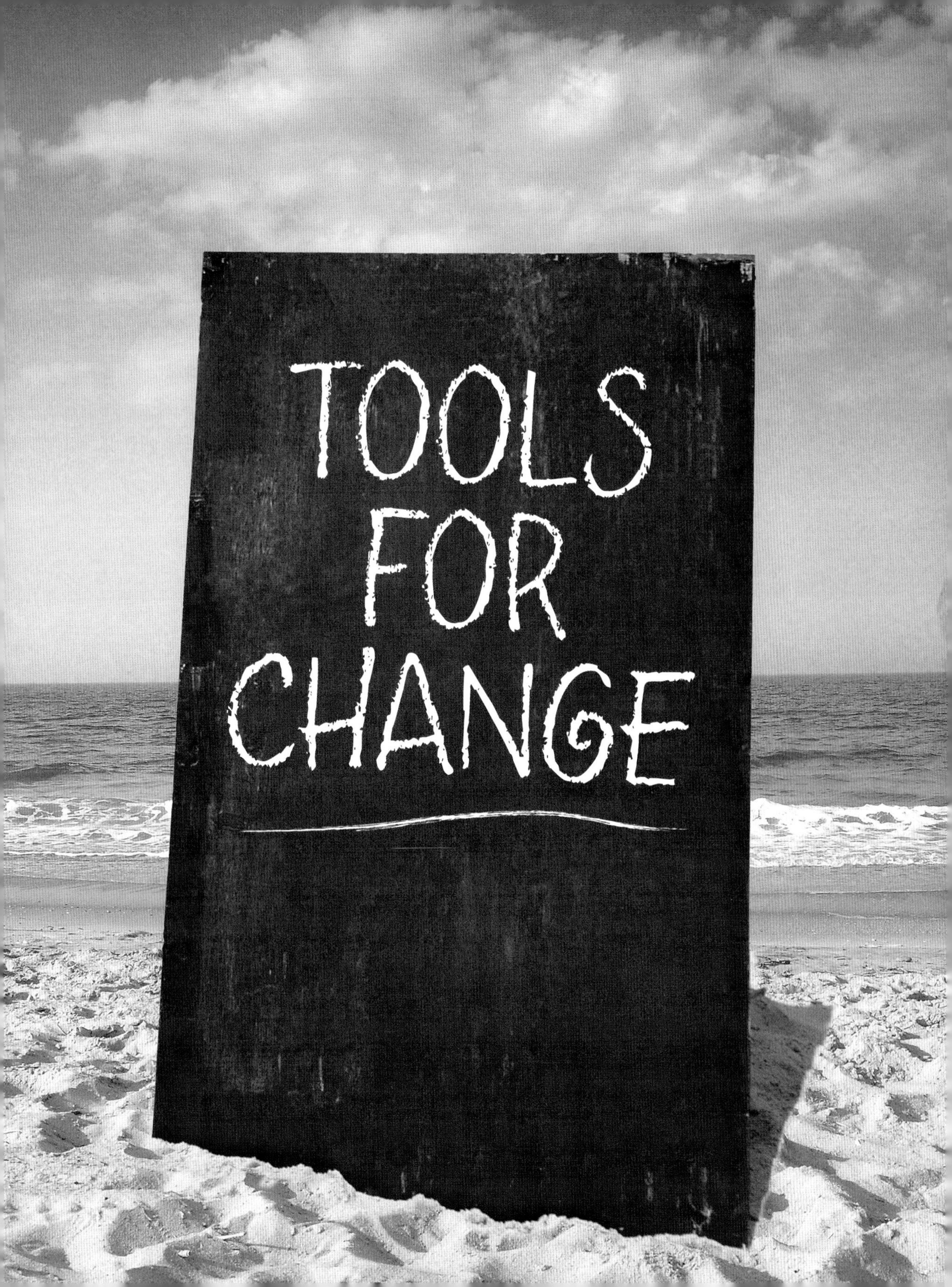
TOOLS
FOR
CHANGE

Menu Plans

Feeling good and looking great can be achieved through a healthy lifestyle consisting of regular exercise and clean eating. We've devised a three-week meal plan to keep you on track and feeling motivated. Recipes for the meals listed here can be found within the 'Clean Eating' section of this book. We also have a few tips to help you along the way.

1. Shop smart. Choose what you buy carefully. Go for organic or local produce, and sustainable and ethical meat, poultry and seafood. We know that sometimes finding the money to buy premium produce is difficult, so just stay mindful and do what you can. We are what we eat, so don't be quick, cheap or fake.

2. Keep your fluids up. Water is so vital to our health and wellbeing. It truly is our detoxification tool, flushing waste from our bodies. When possible, filter your water for increased alkalising effects. Remember: coffee, juices and soft drinks do not contribute to your daily water consumption.

3. Snack right. You might feel like snacking throughout the day between meals, and we recommend you stay fuelled, to avoid excess weight gain and so you won't be tempted to reach for a naughty snack. Have some activated almonds, a natural protein shake or fresh fruit on hand for when you get peckish.

4. Be prepared. Plan ahead for the week's meals. Sit down on a Sunday and jot down what ingredients you need for each meal, then get shopping and prepare yourself for a week of good nutrition.

5. Keep a food diary. You'll stick to a healthy eating plan much more easily if you keep a food diary. By jotting down what you eat and when, you get a true idea of your daily habits, and it can make you aware of bad habits.

6. Make it fun. Get some friends together and share the workload. Perhaps you can take it in turns cooking our recipes together at each other's houses. You are more likely to stick to a healthy living plan if you have someone to do it with.

7. Treat yourself. Sometimes to stay on track you need to treat yourself. We recommend having just one cheat meal per week. It will curb your cravings and keep you on the right path for the rest of the time.

Week One

	Breakfast	Lunch	Dinner
Monday	Amaranth and Chia Porridge	Chilli Lamb and Quinoa Salad with Roast Beetroot, Feta and Toasted Pine Nuts	Crispy-skin Ocean Trout, Pea Puree, Sweet Potato Discs, Fennel and Zucchini Salad with Lime Aioli
Tuesday	Banana and Quinoa Porridge	Spicy Kangaroo Burgers Stacked with Sweet Potato Fritters and Sautéed Kale	Pecan-crusted Tuna with a Superfood Pink Grapefruit and Black Quinoa Salad
Wednesday	Surf-side Granola with Raspberries	Zucchini Linguine with Poached Rainbow Trout	Lamb Cutlets with a Zucchini, Pea and Mint Salad
Thursday	Paleo Parfait	Luke and Scott's Niçoise	Dukkah Kangaroo with Freekeh, Roast Cauliflower and Pomegranate Salad and Sweet Potato Discs
Friday	Perfect Poached Eggs with Sautéed Kale on Sprouted Toast	Salmon, Cherry Tomato and Kale Frittata	Chilli Salt Scotch Fillet with Avocado and a Pear and Rocket Salad
Saturday	Shakshuka with Crispy Bacon	Crispy-skin Barramundi with Mango Relish	Sweet Potato Gnocchi with Pounded Walnut Sauce
Sunday	Coconut Pancakes with Blueberry Coulis	Quinoa and Sweetcorn Fritters with Avocado and Tomato Salsa	Adobo Roast Chicken, Red Cabbage and Lime Slaw and Chimichurri

Week Two

	Breakfast	Lunch	Dinner
Monday	Banana and Quinoa Porridge	Luke and Scott's Niçoise	Lamb Cutlets with a Zucchini, Pea and Mint Salad
Tuesday	Paleo Parfait	Salmon, Cherry Tomato and Kale Frittata	Crispy-skin Ocean Trout, Pea Puree, Sweet Potato Discs, Fennel and Zucchini Salad with Lime Aioli
Wednesday	Oat and Chia Porridge	Chilli Lamb and Quinoa Salad with Roast Beetroot, Feta and Toasted Pine Nuts	Pecan-crusted Tuna with a Superfood Pink Grapefruit and Black Quinoa Salad
Thursday	Surf-side Granola with Raspberries	Spicy Kangaroo Burgers Stacked with Sweet Potato Fritters and Sautéed Kale	Adobo Roast Chicken, Red Cabbage and Lime Slaw and Chimichurri
Friday	Perfect Poached Eggs with Avocado and Crispy Bacon on Sprouted Toast	Zucchini Linguine with Poached Rainbow Trout	Sweet Potato Gnocchi with Pounded Walnut Sauce
Saturday	Coconut Pancakes with Coconut Yoghurt	Quinoa and Sweetcorn Fritters with Avocado and Tomato Salsa	Chilli Salt Scotch Fillet with Avocado and a Pear and Rocket Salad
Sunday	Shakshuka with Crispy Bacon	Crispy-skin Barramundi with Mango Relish	Dukkah Kangaroo with Freekeh, Roast Cauliflower and Pomegranate Salad and Sweet Potato Discs

Week Three

	Breakfast	Lunch	Dinner
Monday	Paleo Parfait	Zucchini Linguine with Poached Rainbow Trout	Sweet Potato Gnocchi with Pounded Walnut Sauce
Tuesday	Amaranth and Chia Porridge	Crispy-skin Barramundi with Mango Relish	Lamb Cutlets with a Zucchini, Pea and Mint Salad
Wednesday	Perfect Poached Eggs with Smoked Salmon on Sprouted Toast	Quinoa and Sweetcorn Fritters with Avocado and Tomato Salsa	Pecan-crusted Tuna with a Superfood Pink Grapefruit and Black Quinoa Salad
Thursday	Banana and Quinoa Porridge	Luke and Scott's Niçoise	Dukkah Kangaroo with Freekeh, Roast Cauliflower and Pomegranate Salad and Sweet Potato Discs
Friday	Surf-side Granola with Mixed Berries	Chilli Lamb and Quinoa Salad with Roast Beetroot, Feta and Toasted Pine Nuts	Adobo Roast Chicken, Red Cabbage and Lime Slaw and Chimichurri
Saturday	Shakshuka with Crispy Bacon	Salmon, Cherry Tomato and Kale Frittata	Chilli Salt Scotch Fillet with Avocado and a Pear and Rocket Salad
Sunday	Coconut Pancakes with Blueberry Coulis	Spicy Kangaroo Burgers Stacked with Sweet Potato Fritters and Sautéed Kale	Crispy-skin Ocean Trout, Pea Puree, Sweet Potato Discs, Fennel and Zucchini Salad with Lime Aioli

Fitness Plans

There are many different ways to structure a work-out session. You might decide how long you want to work out for, the number of repetitions you want to do, or what we call the 'rate of perceived exertion' (how buggered you feel) at the end of the session.

To prescribe an accurate and effective program requires screening and fitness-testing, and we strongly recommend that you see a qualified professional before you embark on a new training regimen, to determine just how hard you can safely push yourself. In the absence of screening and fitness-testing, we suggest that you perform as many reps as you can and stop one or two reps prior to fatigue setting in (at which point your form will diminish). Count the number of reps you do each time, as this will become your benchmark for your next set.

Every session should begin with a thorough warm-up incorporating all the major joints – knee, hip, spine, shoulder and elbow. The warm-up should take around 5 minutes and can include:

- jogging on the spot
- star jumps
- high knees (lifting your knees up to your chest, one at a time)
- rotation/range-of-motion exercises for all the joints (start small and slow and increase the range and the speed over 20 to 30 seconds)
- walking lunges
- a gentle run (1 to 2 minutes).

The aim of the warm-up is to literally warm up the fluid in the joints, get blood flowing to the muscles and raise your heart rate. It should bring on a light sweat.

Unless we specify otherwise, try to complete as many continuous reps of each exercise as you can before moving on to the next, or, in the case of a static exercise like a plank, just stop 2 to 5 seconds before fatigue sets in.

Try to complete as many routines as you can each week. The routines are fairly short, so they're perfect for the time-poor among us.

Week One

DAY ONE
Squats
Mountain climbers
Kneel to standing (2 minutes)
Frogs (1 minute)
Repeat 4 to 6 times

DAY TWO
Run (15 to 20 minutes – cover as much
   distance as you can)
Elephant walk (2 minutes)
Plank
Repeat once

DAY THREE
Push-ups
Flutter kicks
Sprawls
Reverse lunges
Repeat 3 to 5 times

DAY FOUR
Squats
Thrusters
Straight arm/leg opposite toe taps
Elephant walk (2 minutes)
Repeat 3 to 5 times

DAY FIVE
Stair work (15 to 20 minutes)
Frogs (1 minute)
Flutter kicks
Plank

DAY SIX
Squats
Sprawls
Mountain climbers
Elephant walk (2 minutes)
Repeat 3 to 5 times

DAY SEVEN
Rest

Week Two

DAY ONE
Roll-back with kick-ups (at least 1 minute)
Box lunges
Frogs (1 minute)
Push-ups
Straight arm/leg opposite toe taps

DAY TWO
Run (15 to 20 minutes – cover as much
   distance as you can)
Elephant walk (2 minutes)
Sprawls
Flutter kicks
Plank

DAY THREE
Split lunges
Thrusters
Plank
Straight arm/leg opposite toe taps
Repeat 4 to 6 times

DAY FOUR
Kettlebell swings
Box lunges
Mountain climbers
Repeat 4 to 6 times

DAY FIVE
Stair work (15 to 20 minutes)
Squats
Push-ups
Elephant walk
Plank

DAY SIX
Split lunges
Roll-back with kick-ups
Thrusters
Sprawls
Repeat 4 to 6 times

DAY SEVEN
Rest

Week Three

Kettlebell squats with overhead press
Mountain climbers
Roll-back with kick-ups
Thrusters
Plank
Repeat 4 to 6 times

DAY TWO
Bounding (15 to 20 minutes – on a flat
  surface, or, even better, on stairs)
Ultimate push-ups
Elephant walk (2 minutes)
Flutter kicks

DAY THREE
Kettlebell swings
Elephant walk
Split lunges
Sprawls
Straight arm/leg opposite toe taps
Repeat 4 to 6 times

DAY FOUR
Box lunges
Frogs (1 minute)
Squat jumps
Plank
Repeat 4 to 6 times

DAY FIVE
Bounding (15 to 20 minutes)
Kettlebell swings
Sprawls
Ultimate push-ups
Plank

DAY SIX
Roll-back with kick-ups
Squat jumps
Mountain climbers
Flutter kicks
Straight arm/leg opposite toe taps
Squats with overhead press

DAY SEVEN
Rest

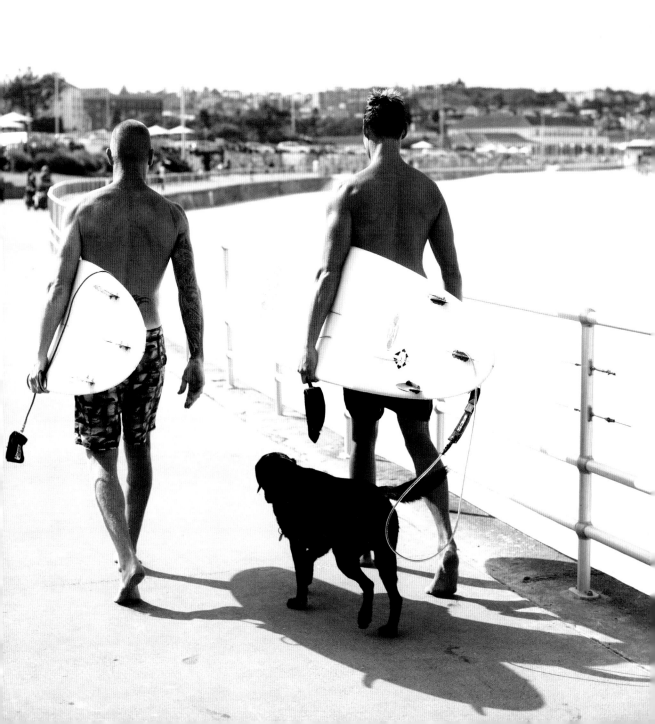

Index

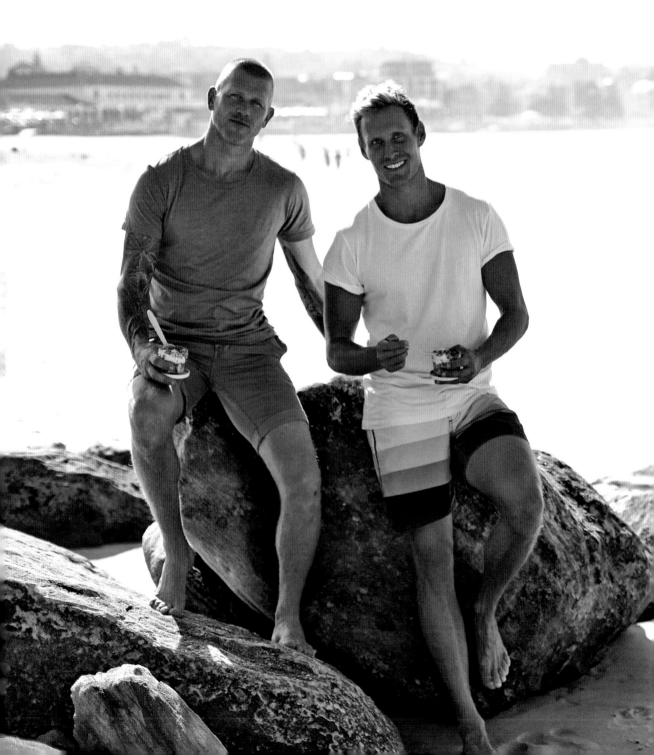

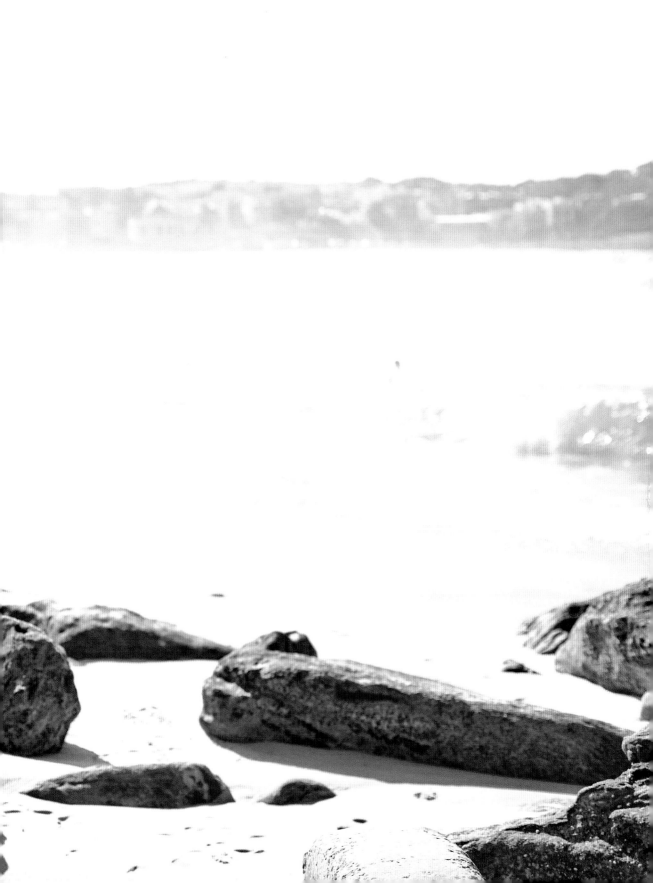

Luke would like to thank ...

It is overwhelmingly wonderful to have the opportunity to thank the people who have helped make one of my dreams come true. So, here goes (feels like an Oscar speech) ...

To Rikkie Proost, the creator and executive producer of the hit series *My Kitchen Rules*: your vision, creativity and commitment to such an amazing program gave us the perfect platform to launch our personal brand and share our beliefs with a massive audience. To Matt Apps: you played a huge role in the journey we took from the day we auditioned to the air date of the finale. Without such an arena to cook the food we are passionate about, this book would not be here today. To the many other producers, assistants, make-up and crew who worked on *MKR*, we wouldn't have been able to be the Bondi Boys had it not been for your friendship, hard work and dedication.

Pete and Manu: at times you were the scariest guys in the world, as we stood there shaking, one of us always crying, waiting for our critique. But you truly got the best out of us and offered us a friendship that we didn't expect. And your talent, experience and professionalism gave us the ability to write and cook the way we do today.

To my family, friends and clients: wow! You are patient, giving and loving. I was gone from my everyday life. I couldn't work, couldn't sleep at home, and often couldn't keep my eyes open after massive days of filming. And just as soon as I was back in real life I started writing this book and again had my focus elsewhere. Thanks for sticking by me through thick and thin and allowing me to create what will be the start of many books to inspire the world to be a happier, healthier place.

To the entire crew working on this, our baby. Without our commissioning editor Robert believing in us from before we had even cooked a single dish on the show, we would not be here today. He took a gamble on two guys from the beach, just trying to cook some healthy food, and his vision, creativity and hard work has landed us with a fantastic publisher. He is to be commended. As is our editor Kate, who kept us on time with consistent deadlines, but always with such gentle and kind encouragement.

To our fabulous food team, stylist and photographer: Tracey, Trish and Steve. This truly is the dream team. From on location to in the kitchen studio, they were the magic makers, making our food look better than I ever have while showing a passion and a belief in us that actually brought tears to my eyes. They captured our best side. And, of course, thanks to our models also, who very generously donated their time to help us with this beautiful book. Thanks, guys, truly inspiring.

I dedicate this, my first book, to my biggest fans: my beautiful mum and dad. Life hasn't always been easy, and it can throw us curve balls, but you have believed in me from day one and, most importantly, you've never ever given up on me or my dreams. Thank you. I love you both.

Scott would like to thank ...

Getting to this point in my life has been a consequence of hard work, perseverance and good fortune. Good fortune to have people in my life that have been supportive and encouraging throughout. It has long been a goal of mine to spread the health and fitness message far and wide, and I would like to mention Channel 7 and *MKR* for giving Luke and I the opportunity to do that – in particular Manu Feildel, Pete Evans and Rikkie Proost. Also, a special thanks to my mum and sister for their continued support and love. I dedicate this book to my late father, Richard.

I would also like to say a massive thanks to the creative team involved in making our project come to fruition. You all made this a pleasurable experience and one which we would love to repeat. A big thanks to the A-team: Steve Brown (photographer), Trish Heagerty (food stylist), Tracey Meharg (foodie), Jessica Luca (production), Kate Stevens (editor) for keeping us in check, and of course to the wonderful Robert Watkins (publisher) for having faith in us from the start. We couldn't have done it without everyone's hard work, enthusiasm and passion. Love you guys!

A special thanks to Earth Food Store at Bondi, and to the fab models, Tilly, Liv and Flo – thanks for your patience!

Also, thanks and respect to Spring Court Australia and Academy Brand.

GET IN TOUCH WITH LUKE:

www.trainerluke.com

Tweet me:
@bondiPT

Instagram me:
@trainer_luke

Facebook me:
www.facebook.com/thebondipt

GET IN TOUCH WITH SCOTT:

www.scottgoodingfitness.com.au

Tweet me:
@ScottyFit

Instagram me:
@scottyfit

GET IN TOUCH WITH LUKE AND SCOTT:

www.lukeandscott.com

Tweet us:
@LukeandScottMKR

Facebook us:
www.facebook.com/lukeandscottmkr

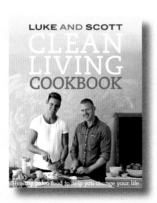

**CLEAN LIVING COOKBOOK
available February 2014**